PORTABLE

50

HERBAL REMEDIES
For DIABETES

Recipes that Support Healthy Living and help with Disease Management - particularly for Type 2 Diabetes.

By **CYNTHIA LEONARD**

TABLE OF CONTENTS

INTRODUCTION

Understanding Diabetes And The Benefits of Herbs and Herbal Spices In Managing Type 2 Diabetes.

Elevated blood sugar (glucose) levels are a hallmark of type 2 diabetes, a chronic illness brought on by either insulin resistance or inadequate pancreatic insulin secretion. Its prevalence and related problems make it a major worldwide health issue.

Several tactics are used to manage type 2 diabetes, such as medication, lifestyle changes and sometimes insulin treatment.

The potential advantages of using herbs and herbal spices in the treatment of diabetes have attracted increasing attention in recent years. Certain herbs and spices have shown potential in assisting with blood sugar regulation and enhancing insulin sensitivity, while research in this area is still continuing.

Here are few instances:

Cinnamon: Research indicates that cinnamon may help decrease blood sugar and enhance insulin sensitivity. In addition to having substances that resemble insulin, it may also slow down the digestion of carbs, resulting in more stable blood sugar levels.

Fenugreek: By slowing down the absorption of carbs, soluble fibre found in fenugreek seeds may help control blood sugar levels. They could also lower fasting blood sugar levels and increase insulin sensitivity.

Ginger: Due to its anti-inflammatory and antioxidant qualities, ginger may help reduce blood sugar and enhance insulin sensitivity. Also, it could protect the pancreas, which is in charge of making insulin.

Turmeric: Curcumin, the main ingredient in turmeric, has been researched for possible anti-diabetic properties. It could lessen inflammation, raise insulin sensitivity and decrease blood sugar.

Ginseng: Research has been done on the potential benefits of both American and Asian ginseng for lowering blood sugar and improving insulin sensitivity. To establish their efficacy and establish the right dose, additional study is necessary.

Bitter melon: Compounds in bitter melon may enhance insulin secretion and glucose utilisation, resulting in lowered blood sugar levels. It is often used in conventional medicine to treat diabetes.

Basil: Holy basil, also known as tulsi, has been shown to have anti-diabetic benefits, such as raising insulin production and lowering blood sugar levels. Also, it could aid in preventing diabetic complications including kidney damage.

There is potential for certain herbs and spices to help manage type 2 diabetes, it is important to utilise them as part of a complete treatment plan under a doctor's supervision.

While they may supplement current treatments and improve general health and well-being, they are not intended to take the place of conventional medical care.

Furthermore, each person may react differently to these herbs, so it's important to keep a careful eye on your blood sugar levels while using them.

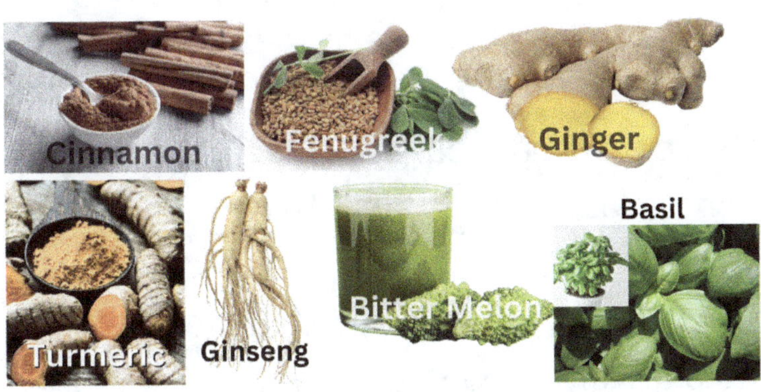

PART 1:

Types of Diabetes Friendly Herbs

A list of 50 herbs that have been traditionally used or studied for their potential benefits in managing diabetes below:

Ginseng: May help improve blood sugar control and insulin sensitivity.

Cinnamon: Some studies suggest it may help lower blood sugar levels.

Fenugreek: Can help lower blood sugar levels and improve insulin function.

Bitter melon: Contains compounds that may mimic insulin and help lower blood sugar levels.

Gymnema: Known as the **"sugar destroyer,"** it may help lower blood sugar levels and improve insulin function.

Aloe vera: May have blood sugar-lowering effects, but more research is needed.

Berberine: Found in several plants like goldenseal and barberry, it may help lower blood sugar levels.

Holy Basil (Tulsi): Can help lower blood sugar levels and improve insulin secretion.

Turmeric: Contains curcumin, which may help improve insulin sensitivity.

Ginger: May improve insulin sensitivity and reduce inflammation.

Dandelion: May help regulate blood sugar levels.

Chamomile: May have potential benefits for lowering blood sugar levels.

Licorice Root: Some studies suggest it may help lower blood sugar levels, but it should be used cautiously due to potential side effects.

Milk thistle: May help improve blood sugar control and protect the liver.

Bilberry: Contains compounds that may help improve insulin sensitivity.

Garlic: May have benefits for blood sugar and cholesterol levels.

Nettle: May help regulate blood sugar levels.

Sage: May improve insulin sensitivity and lower blood sugar levels.

Oregano: Contains compounds that may help lower blood sugar levels.

Parsley: May have potential benefits for lowering blood sugar levels.

Rosemary: Contains compounds that may improve insulin sensitivity.

Peppermint: May help improve digestion and potentially aid in blood sugar control.

Ginger: Contains compounds that may improve insulin sensitivity.

Black seed (*Nigella sativa*): May have blood sugar-lowering effects.

Eucalyptus: May help improve blood sugar control.

Juniper berries: May have potential benefits for lowering blood sugar levels.

Saffron: Some studies suggest it may help improve insulin sensitivity.

Cat's claw: May help regulate blood sugar levels.

Clove: Contains compounds that may help improve insulin function.

Guggul: May have potential benefits for improving insulin sensitivity.

Yarrow: May help regulate blood sugar levels.

Burdock Root: May have potential benefits for blood sugar control.

Goat's rue: Traditionally used for diabetes management, but scientific evidence is limited.

Prickly Pear Cactus: Some studies suggest it may help lower blood sugar levels.

Mistletoe: May have potential benefits for blood sugar control.

Siberian ginseng: May help improve insulin sensitivity.

American ginseng: Similar to Siberian ginseng, it may help improve insulin sensitivity.

Hawthorn: May have potential benefits for cardiovascular health in diabetes.

Ginger root: Contains compounds that may improve insulin sensitivity.

Momordica charantia (**Bitter melon**): May help lower blood sugar levels.

Echinacea: May have potential benefits for immune health in diabetes management.

Fenugreek seeds: May help improve insulin sensitivity and lower blood sugar levels.

Hibiscus: Some studies suggest it may help regulate blood sugar levels.

Mango leaves: Traditionally used for managing diabetes, but scientific evidence is limited.

Okra: Contains compounds that may help lower blood sugar levels.

Soybean: May have potential benefits for improving insulin sensitivity.

Astragalus: Some studies suggest it may help improve insulin sensitivity.

Rhodiola: May have potential benefits for stress management, which could indirectly affect blood sugar levels.

Ashwagandha: May help improve insulin sensitivity and lower blood sugar levels.

Chaste Tree: Some studies suggest it may help improve insulin sensitivity.

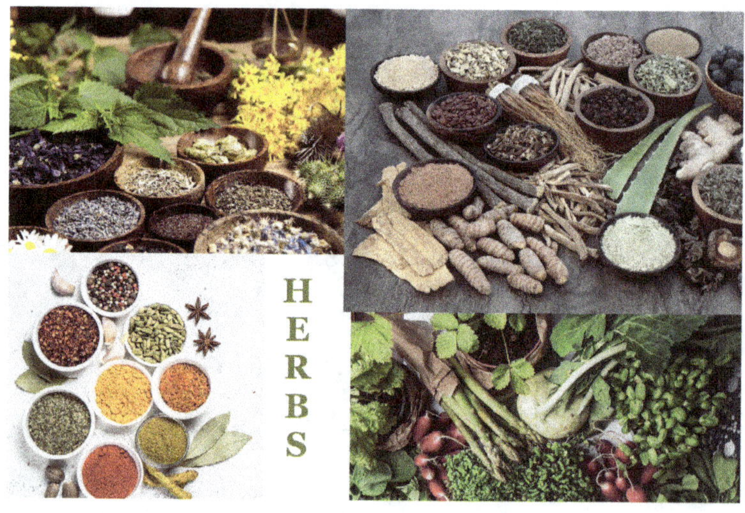

Variety Of Herbs

PART 2

50 Herbal Remedies Recipes

Here's a list of **50** herbal remedy recipes that may complement a diabetes diet and management plan. These recipes include various herbs and ingredients.

CINNAMON TEA

Ingredients:

- 1 teaspoon of ground cinnamon or 2 cinnamon sticks.
- 2 glasses of water
- Sugar or honey *(optional; taste and adjust)*
- Cream or milk *(to taste, optional)*

Instruction:

In a saucepan or kettle, start by bringing two cups of water to a boil. As the water heats up, have your cinnamon sticks ready.

To aid release the flavour, split the cinnamon sticks into tiny pieces *if using them.*

When the water is boiling, add the ground cinnamon or cinnamon sticks to the saucepan.

After bringing the heat to low, simmer the cinnamon in the water for 10 to 15 minutes. This permits the taste to seep into the water.

After boiling for a few minutes, take the pot off of the hob and allow it to cool somewhat.

If you are using ground cinnamon - strain the tea to get rid of any particles or cinnamon sticks.

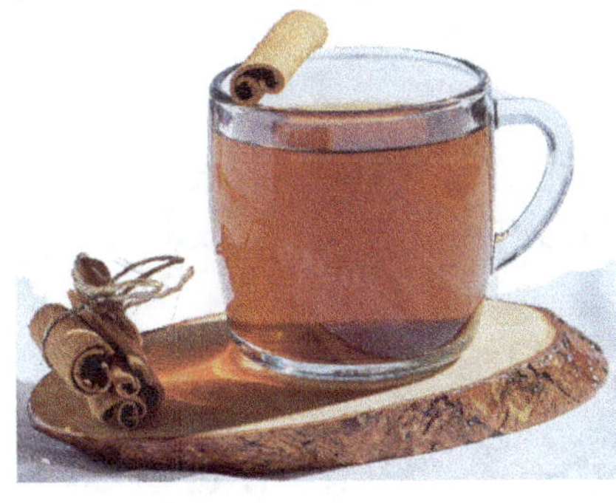

You may add honey or sugar to taste to sweeten your cinnamon tea if you'd like.

To get a creamier texture, you may also add milk or cream.

Serve hot cinnamon tea after giving it a good stir.

GINGER LEMONADE

Ingredients:

- Juice from 1 cup of freshly squeezed lemons *(approximately four to six)*.
- Half a cup of granulated sugar, or to taste
- 4 glasses of cold water
- Two to three teaspoons of freshly grated Ginger.
- Cubes of ice
- Slices of lemon and fresh mint are **optional** garnishes.

Instruction:

Add one cup of water and the grated ginger to a small pot and simmer for about 5 minutes on medium heat after bringing to a boil.

Take it off the stove and give it some time to cool.

To extract the ginger pulp, strain the infusion of water with ginger using a cheesecloth or fine mesh strainer and save the liquid in a measuring cup or basin.

Throw away the pulped ginger.

Pour the remaining 3 cups of cold water, sugar and freshly squeezed lemon juice into a large pitcher. Until the sugar dissolves, stir.

Fill the pitcher with the infusion of ginger and whisk to mix.

If desired, taste the lemonade and add extra sugar or lemon juice to modify the sweetness or bitterness.

Chill the lemonade in the refrigerator for at least an hour.

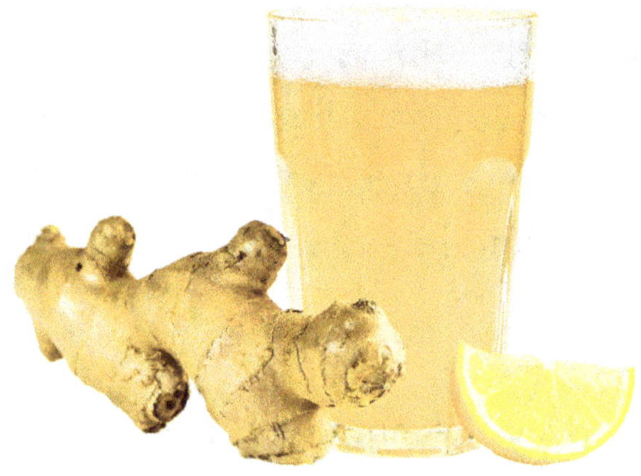

Pour the ginger lemonade into glasses with ice cubes. *If preferred,* garnish with fresh mint leaves and lemon slices.

FENUGREEK SEED SPROUTS

Ingredients:

- 1/4 cup of seeds for fenugreek
- Water

Instruction:

Allow the Seeds to Soak: After taking out 1/4 cup of fenugreek seeds, give them a good rinse under running water.

Pour the seeds into a basin and add just enough water to completely submerge them.

Soak the seeds for 8 to 12 hours, *if possible,* preferably overnight. This will cause the seeds to become softer and start the sprouting process.

Empty and Wash: Use a strainer or colander to remove the seeds' water after soaking.

To remove any last bits of dirt, give the seeds another thorough rinse under fresh water.

Move to a Container for Sprouting: Place the seeds in a sprouting container once they have been soaked and cleaned. Use any sprout-safe container, such as a tray or sprouting jar.

Make sure there is enough drainage in the container to avoid waterlogging.

To Plant the Seeds: *The container should be kept out of direct sunlight and in a well-ventilated location.*

Make sure the seeds are damp but not soggy by rinsing them with water two to three times a day.

Depending on the environment and the desired length of sprouts, continue this technique for about 2-4 days. Sprouts of fenugreek usually reach a length of 1-2 inches.

To gather the sprouts: *You may harvest the sprouts once they reach the required length.*

Store or Utilise: Fenugreek sprouts should be used right away in your preferred salad, sandwich or stir-fry dishes. The sprouts should be kept in the refrigerator in an airtight container if you won't be using them straight away.

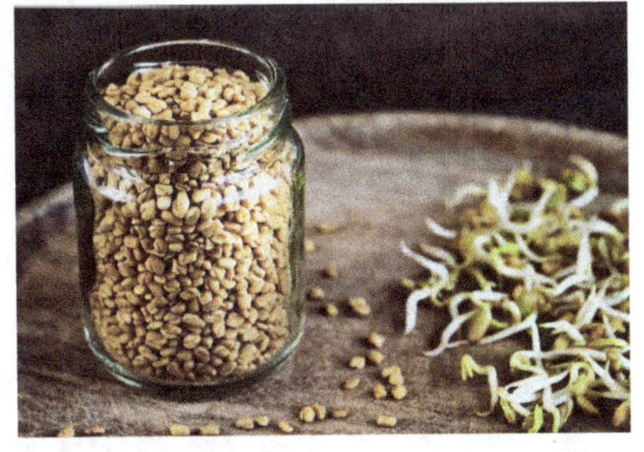

They ought to be kept for two or three days. Savour the sprouts of your homegrown fenugreek seeds.

Optional Tip: To aid with drainage and washing, some people like to cover the sprouting container

TURMERIC MILK

Ingredients:

- Two cups of milk *(you may use any kind of milk, such as coconut, almond or cow's milk)*.
- One teaspoon of powdered turmeric *(or grated fresh turmeric root)*
- half a teaspoon of cinnamon powder
- 1/4 tsp freshly grated Ginger or ground Ginger.

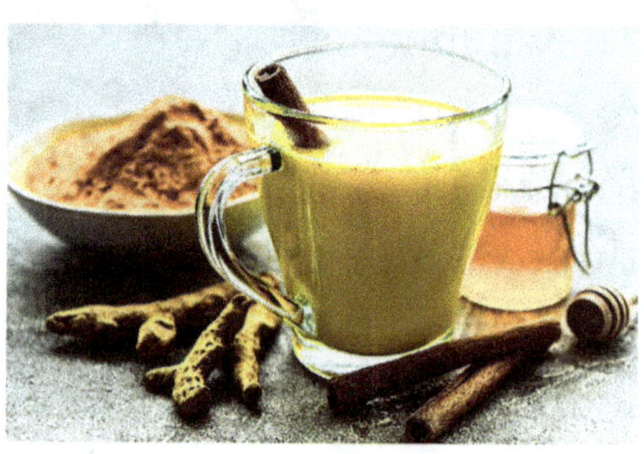

- A dash of black pepper, *if desired*

- Add sweetener *(sugar, maple syrup or honey)* to taste.
- A little bit of extractive vanilla *(optional)*

Instruction:

Transfer the milk into a small saucepan and set it over medium heat on the stove.

To the milk, add the ground turmeric, ginger, cinnamon and black pepper.

Mix the ingredients well by whisking them together.

Simmer the milk slowly for around 5 minutes, stirring from time to time. *Take care not to allow it to boil.*

After taking the pot from the stove, let the milk with turmeric cool somewhat.

Stir in your preferred sweetener until it dissolves. *The quantity of sweetness may be changed to suit your tastes.*

For added taste, stir in a little amount of vanilla essence, *if using.*

To get rid of any lumps or big bits of spice - strain the turmeric milk through a fine mesh strainer *(you may skip this step if you don't mind the texture).*

Transfer the strained turmeric milk into heated mugs or glasses.

If you'd like, you may garnish by adding a little additional ground cinnamon on top.

Savour your relaxing and warm turmeric milk.
It is ideal as a soothing beverage at any time of day or just before bed.

BITTER MELON STIR-FRY

Ingredients:

- One bitter, medium-sized melon
- One tablespoon of cooking oil, such as peanut or vegetable oil.
- 2 minced garlic cloves
- 1 little onion, cut into slices
- 1 little tomato, chopped *(optional)*
- A quarter of a pound of thinly sliced pork *(optional, for flavour)*
- 2 tsp soy sauce
- 1 spoonful of sauce for Oysters
- Half a teaspoon of sugar
- Salt and pepper.
- Fresh chilli or red chilli flakes *(optional, for extra spiciness)*

Instruction:
Cut the bitter melon in half lengthwise to prepare it.

Using a spoon, remove the seeds and pith.

Cut the sour melon into slender half-moons. *If you'd like*, you may also cut it into circles.

If using pork, marinade it for 10 to 15 minutes with a little amount of soy sauce, salt and pepper.

In a wok or big pan, heat the cooking oil over medium-high heat. Add the onion slices and minced garlic.

Sauté until they become transparent and aromatic.

Add the pork to the pan and stir-fry it until it's cooked through, *if using*.

Sliced bitter melon should be added to the wok. Stir-fry for 3 to 5 minutes or until it becomes somewhat tender.

Add the sugar, oyster sauce, soy sauce, sliced tomato and a dash of salt and pepper. Mix well to blend.

Cook the bitter melon for a further 3 to 5 minutes or until it reaches the desired level of softness.

You may cover the wok and let it steam for a few minutes if you want it softer. **If necessary**, taste and adjust the seasoning.

 Add fresh chilli or red chilli flakes, depending on how spicy you want it to be.

When finished, take off the heat and serve hot with steamed rice.

GINSENG CHICKEN SOUP

A classic Korean meal noted for its nutritious and revitalising qualities is ginseng chicken soup. *This is a simple recipe for Soup with Ginseng Chicken:*

Ingredients:

- 1 whole chicken, weighing around 3–4 pounds.
- Eight glasses of water
- 10–12 peeled garlic cloves
- 10–12 jujubes or dried red dates
- 10–12 dried or fresh ginseng roots
- One medium-sized onion, cut in half and stripped
- 3 chopped green onions

- Salt and pepper.
- **Optional**: One cup of glutinous rice, also referred to as sweet rice, steeped for one hour.

Instruction:

After giving the whole chicken a good rinse in cold water, trim off any extra fat.

Before beginning, let the sweet rice soak in water for about 1 hour.

Bring 8 cups of water to a boil in a big saucepan.

Put the whole chicken in the water that is boiling. To get rid of any contaminants, boil it for around 5 minutes.

Once the chicken is out of the saucepan, dispose of the water. Use cold water to rinse the chicken.

After cleaning, pour in some new water. Once again, bring it to a boil.

Re-add the cleaned chicken to the boiling water pot.

Add the onion, ginseng roots, dried red dates, cloves of garlic and soaked sweet rice, *if using.*

Once the chicken is thoroughly cooked and soft, reduce the heat to medium-low and simmer the soup for 1 to 2 hours.

While cooking, skim off any froth that comes to the top.

Season the soup to taste with salt and pepper about half an hour before it's done.

Take the saucepan off of the hob once the chicken has cooked through and the flavours have combined.

Garnish the heated soup with finely chopped green onions.

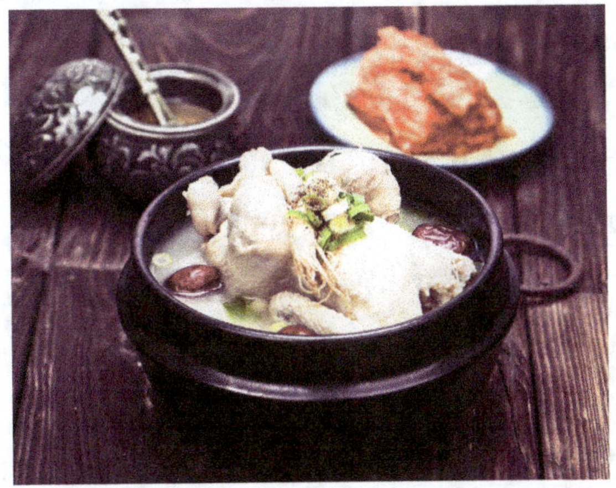

Traditionally, the soup is served with a chunk of chicken, red dates, cloves of garlic and some ginseng roots.

CILANTRO LIME QUINOA

Ingredients:

- 1 cup of quinoa
- 2 cups of veggie broth or water
- One lime, juiced
- 1/4 cup of freshly chopped cilantro
- Salt and pepper.

Instructions:

To get rid of any bitter coating, rinse the quinoa in a fine-mesh strainer under cold water and put it in a medium pot with either water or vegetable broth.

Heat to a boil on a medium-high heat setting.

After the quinoa begins to boil, lower the heat to a simmer - cover and cook for 15 to 20 minutes or until the quinoa is tender and the liquid has been absorbed then using a fork, fluff.

After cooking, transfer the quinoa to a mixing bowl.

Stir the quinoa with the chopped cilantro and freshly squeezed lime juice. Mix everything together.

To taste, add salt and pepper for seasoning.

Warm this up as a side dish or to use as a foundation for your preferred protein and veggies.

ROSEMARY ROASTED VEGETABLES

Vegetables cooked with rosemary form a tasty and aromatic side dish.

Ingredients:

- Mixed veggies, chopped into wedges or pieces *(such as potatoes, carrots, bell peppers, zucchini, onions, etc.)*
- Olive oil
- Salt and pepper.
- Fresh rosemary sprigs, chopped or whole

Instruction:

Set oven temperature to 400°F or 200°C.

Wash and chop the veggies into pieces that are about the same size. This guarantees uniform cooking.

Put the veggies in a big basin for mixing.

Make sure the veggies have a light coating on them when you drizzle them with olive oil.

Just enough oil should be used to help the seasoning and rosemary cling, but not so much that they are submerged in it.

To taste, add salt and pepper to the veggies then make sure the oil and seasoning are applied evenly by giving them a little toss.

Arrange the veggies on a baking sheet so they are in a single layer.

You may line the baking pan with aluminium foil or parchment paper if you don't want them to stick.

Garnish the veggies with chopped rosemary or fresh sprigs of rosemary.

The meal gets a fantastic flavour and perfume from the rosemary.

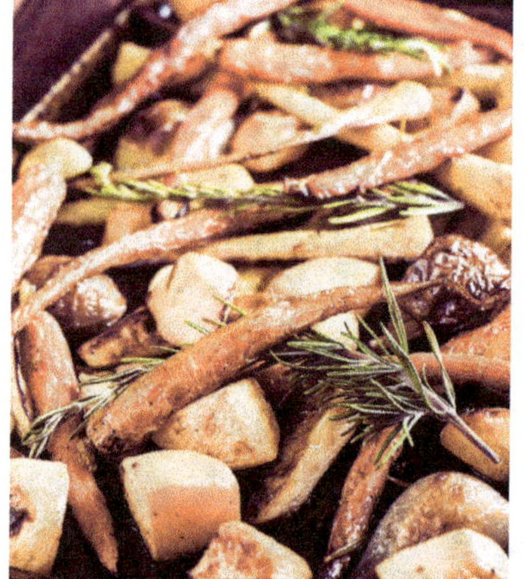

After preheating the oven, place the baking sheet inside and roast the veggies for 25 to 30 minutes or until they are soft and browned, tossing from time to time to ensure equal cooking.

When the veggies are roasted to the doneness you choose, take them out of the oven and serve right away.

BASIL PESTO

Ingredients:

- 2 cups of newly packed basil leaves
- Grate 1/2 cup of Parmesan cheese fresh.
- Half a cup of extra virgin olive oil
- one-third cup walnuts or pine nuts
- 3 minced garlic cloves
- Salt and freshly ground black pepper.

Instruction:

If you're using walnuts or pine nuts, roast them in a small pan over medium heat, turning often, until aromatic and lightly browned.

This should take 5 minutes or so. Leave them to cool.

Combine ingredients: Place the minced garlic, roasted almonds and basil leaves in a food processor. Pulse a few times to chop roughly.

To the mixture in the food processor, add the grated Parmesan cheese.

Blend: Slowly add the olive oil while the food processor is operating. Process the ingredients until it is fully blended and smooth.

To make sure everything is combined evenly, you may need to pause and use a spatula to scrape down the bowl's edges.

Season: Add salt and pepper to taste of the pesto. Keep in mind that Parmesan cheese naturally contains salt, so you may not need much more.

Serve or store: The pesto may be used right away or kept for up to a week in the refrigerator in an airtight container.

You may also freeze it in ice cube trays and store the frozen cubes in a freezer bag for up to several months if you'd want to keep it fresher for longer.

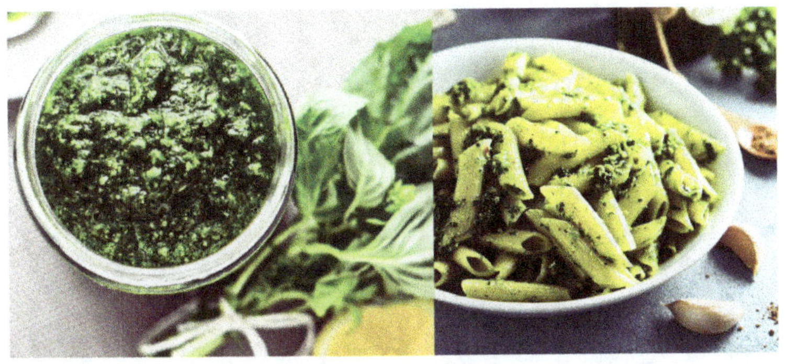

Make your own basil pesto and use it as a pasta sauce, sandwich spread, grilled meat / fish garnish or as a flavour booster added to soups or salads. *There are many options.*

MINTY PEA SOUP

Ingredients:

- 2 tsp olive oil
- one sliced onion
- 2 minced garlic cloves
- 4 cups of broth made with vegetables
- One pound of frozen peas
- Salt and pepper.
- 1/4 cup finely chopped fresh mint leaves
- **Garnish optional:** Sour cream or Greek yoghurt, croutons and mint leaves

Instruction:

In a big saucepan, warm up the olive oil over medium heat. Add chopped onion and minced garlic and cook for approximately 5 minutes or until softened.

After adding the vegetable broth, boil the mixture.

Cook the frozen peas in the saucepan for approximately five minutes or until they are well cooked.

After taking the pot from the stove, let it cool somewhat.

Smooth up the soup using a mixer or immersion blender, working slowly. When combining hot liquids - use caution.

After adding salt and pepper to taste, return the pureed soup to the stove.

Add the chopped mint leaves and cook for a further 2 to 3 minutes to let the flavours combine.

Serve hot, topped with more mint leaves, croutons or a dollop of sour cream or Greek yoghurt, *if you'd like.*

CHAMOMILE RICE PUDDING

Ingredients:

- One cup of rice, Arborio
- 4 glasses of whole milk
- Half a cup of sugar, granulated
- 1 tsp vanilla extract
- 2 tea packets of chamomile
- One-fourth teaspoon salt
- Cinnamon powder *(optional garnish)*

Instruction:

Get the chamomile milk ready by: The milk should be heated in a saucepan over medium heat until it just begins to boil.

Take off the heat and stir in the bags of chamomile tea.

After letting them steep for around 10 minutes, take out the tea bags and squeeze out any extra milk.

Cook the Rice: Put the Arborio rice, sugar, vanilla essence, steeped chamomile milk and salt in a separate, big pot.

Over medium-high heat, bring the mixture to a mild boil while stirring often.

After the mixture reaches a boil, turn down the heat to low and let it simmer uncovered, stirring from time to time. Cook until the rice is soft and the custard has thickened to your preferred consistency, around 25 to 30 minutes.

Serve: Take the rice pudding from the stove and allow it to cool for a few minutes when it reaches the right consistency.

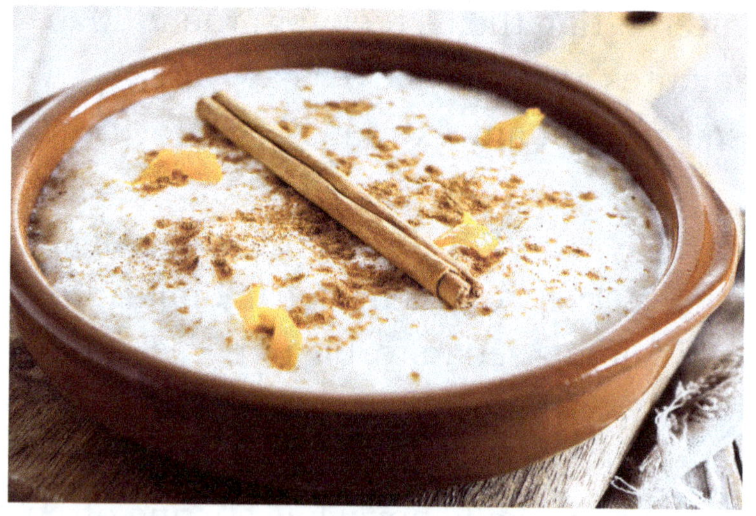

Serve warm or cold, topped, *if like,* with a dusting of ground cinnamon.

Optional: If you would like the rice pudding cold, you may chill it in the refrigerator for a few hours. You may eat it cold or heated.

THYME ROASTED CHICKEN

Ingredients:

- 1 whole chicken, weighing around 3–4 pounds.
- 2 to 3 teaspoons of olive oil
- Salt and pepper.
- 2 to 3 minced garlic cloves
- 2 to 3 fresh thyme sprigs
- One sliced lemon
- Extra herbs, such as sage or rosemary, *are optional.*

Instruction:

Set the oven temperature to 425°F (220°C).

After taking the giblets out of the chicken's cavity, use paper towels to pat the bird dry.

Transfer the chicken to a baking dish or roasting pan.

Drizzle the chicken with olive oil and liberally season it all over, including the cavity, with salt and pepper.

Make sure the minced garlic is properly dispersed throughout the chicken by rubbing it on.

Remove the thyme leaves off the sprigs and gently press them onto the chicken to bind them.

Fill the chicken's cavity with lemon slices and any other herbs you like to use.

If you want to roast the chicken more evenly, tie the legs together with kitchen thread.

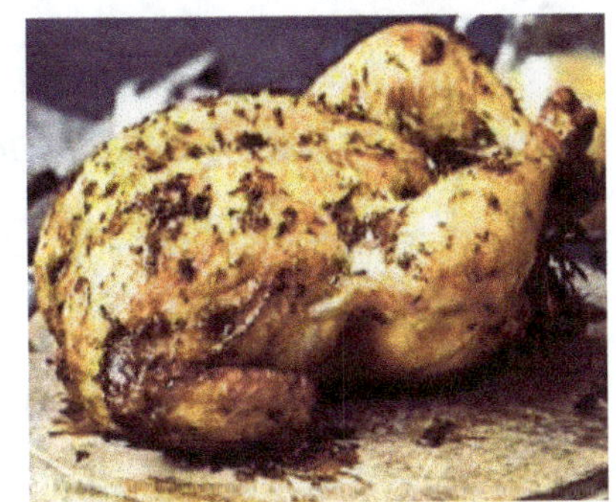

The chicken should be roasted for 1 hour - 1 hour 15 minutes in a preheated oven or until the juices flow clear and an instant-read thermometer put into the thickest portion of the thigh registers 165°F (75°C).

After cooking, take the chicken out of the oven and let it take ten to fifteen minutes to rest before slicing.

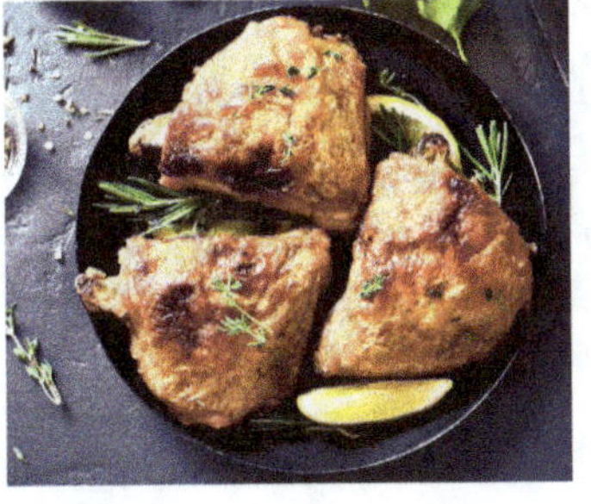

Once carved, serve with your preferred side dishes.

OREGANO TOMATO SALAD

Ingredients:

- Cut into 4 big, ripe tomatoes.
- One-fourth cup of extra virgin olive oil
- Half a tsp balsamic vinegar
- 2 minced garlic cloves
- One tsp of dehydrated oregano
- Salt and pepper.
- Garnish with fresh basil leaves (*optional*).

Instruction:

To create the dressing, combine the olive oil, balsamic vinegar, dried oregano, minced garlic, salt and pepper in a small bowl, then set aside.

After slicing, place the tomatoes on a serving plate.

Make sure the tomatoes are uniformly coated by drizzling them with the dressing.

Give the salad 10 to 15 minutes to marinade so that the flavours may combine.

Garnish with fresh basil leaves just before serving.

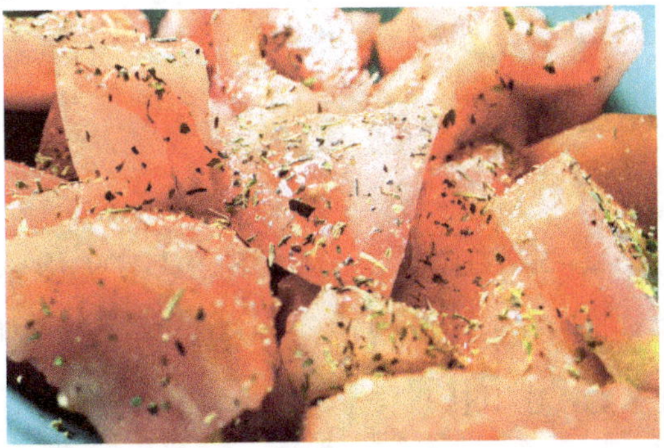

You may serve the Oregano Tomato Salad as a light appetiser or as a side dish.

PARSLEY WALNUT PESTO

Ingredients:

- 1/2 cup roasted walnuts
- 2 cups packed fresh parsley leaves
- 2 peeled garlic cloves
- Grated Parmesan cheese, half a cup
- Half a cup of extra virgin olive oil
- Salt and pepper.

Instruction:

Warm up the walnuts: Set the oven temperature to 350°F (175°C).

Arrange the walnuts in a solitary layer on a baking sheet and bake for about 8 to 10 minutes or until they become aromatic and gently toasted.

They may burn rapidly, so keep an eye on them. When finished, take them out of the oven and let them cool.

Get the ingredients ready: After washing, use a paper towel to gently dry the parsley leaves. Cut the garlic cloves into pieces.

Place the parsley, roasted walnuts, garlic cloves and grated Parmesan cheese in a food processor or blender.

Pulse them a few times - Next, while the food processor is operating, gradually pour in the olive oil until the mixture becomes a thick paste.

To make sure everything is properly blended, you may need to sometimes stop and scrape down the sides of the food processor bowl. Blend until the consistency you want is achieved.

Season: Add salt and pepper to taste, depending on your preferred level of spice. Mix one more time to mix in the spices.

Serve or Store: The pesto may be used right away or kept for up to a week in the refrigerator in an airtight container.

To help prevent oxidation and maintain the pesto's vivid green colour, be sure to lightly coat its surface with olive oil before keeping.

Serving Ideas: For a tasty and fast supper, toss the pesto with your preferred pasta.
- ➤ Spread it over wraps and sandwiches.
- ➤ Serve it as a dip for raw veggies or crackers.
- ➤ Pour it over roasted veggies or grilled meats.

SAGE SWEET POTATO MASH

Ingredients:

- 2 big sweet potatoes, diced and peeled
- 2 tsp butter
- 1/4 cup of milk or more *if necessary*
- One tablespoon of freshly cut sage leaves
- Salt and pepper.

Instruction:

Put the sweet potato cubes in a saucepan and pour water over them. After bringing to a boil, simmer for 15 to 20 minutes or until the sweet potatoes are fork-tender.

After draining, put the sweet potatoes
back in the saucepan.

Sweet potatoes should be added to a
saucepan with butter and mashed with a
potato masher until smooth.

Gradually stir in the milk until the
required consistency is achieved.

Depending on how creamy you want the
mash to be, you may need more or less
milk.

Toss in the
chopped sage
leaves before
adding them to
the sweet
potato mash.

Add salt and pepper to taste and adjust accordingly.

NETTLE LEAF SMOOTHIE

Ingredients:

- 1 cup of fresh nettle leaves *(to prevent stinging, use gloves while handling fresh nettle leaves)*
- One ripe banana
- One cup of **optional** spinach for extra nutrition.
- Half a cup of frozen berries, *such as raspberries, blueberries or strawberries.*
- One tablespoon of **optional** sweetened maple syrup or honey
- One cup of almond milk or any other kind of milk.

- *(Optional, for a cooler smoothie)* Ice cubes

Instruction:

To get rid of any dirt or debris, thoroughly rinse the nettle leaves under cold water.

Take the leaves off of the nettle stalks and blend together the nettle leaves, ripe banana, frozen berries, spinach, honey or maple syrup, *if using,* and almond milk in a blender.

Process at high speed until creamy and smooth.

To get the right consistency, thin down with any extra almond milk or water if the smoothie is too thick.

After tasting the smoothie, add additional honey or maple syrup *if needed* to make it more sweet.

To get a cooler smoothie, add a couple of ice cubes to the blender and process until the mixture is smooth once more.

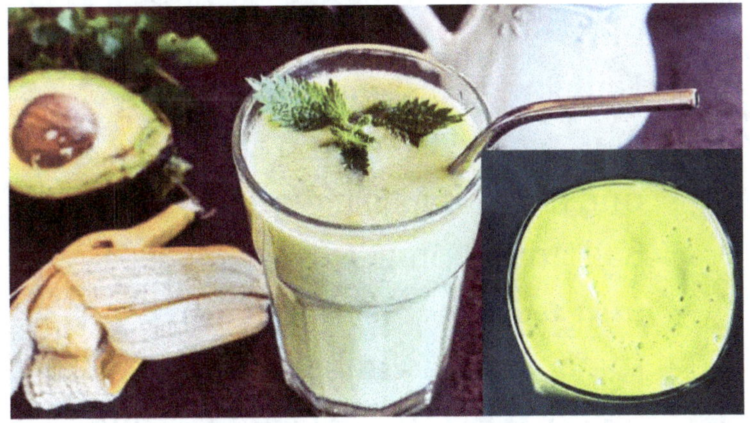

After blending to your desired consistency, transfer the smoothie into glasses and serve right away.

DANDELION GREENS SALAD

Ingredients:

- 4 cups freshly cut and cleaned dandelion greens
- One-fourth cup of extra virgin olive oil
- Half a tsp balsamic vinegar
- One tsp Dijon mustard
- one minced garlic clove
- Salt and pepper.
- **Extra toppings at your discretion:** Cherry tomatoes, cucumber slices, red onion, feta cheese crumbles and toasted nuts *(almonds or walnuts)*

Instruction:

First, give the dandelion greens a good rinse in cold water.

After trimming off any rough stems, cut
the leaves into small pieces.

To remove extra water, spin them in a
salad spinner or pat dry with a fresh
kitchen towel.

Mix the olive oil, balsamic vinegar, Dijon
mustard, minced garlic, salt and pepper in
a small bowl until well combined. *You'll use
this as salad dressing.*

The cut dandelion greens should be put in
a big salad dish. Add any extra toppings,
such as sliced cucumber or cherry
tomatoes, to the bowl as well.

Over the greens and toppings, drizzle the
salad dressing. Toss everything gently
together until the greens are equally
covered with the dressing, using salad
tongs or clean hands *if necessary.*

For extra taste and texture, top the salad with toasted almonds and crumbled feta cheese, *if preferred.*

Serve the salad of dandelion greens right away as a light lunch or as a pleasant side dish.

LAVENDER HONEY GLAZED CARROTS

Ingredients:

- 1 pound (450 grams) of peeled and cut sticks of carrots.
- 2 tsp honey
- One spoonful of butter
- One teaspoon of dehydrated culinary lavender blossoms.
- Salt to taste.
- Ground black pepper *(fresh)*

- Fresh parsley that has been chopped *(optional)*

Instruction:

After peeling, cut the carrots into coins or sticks, depending on your preference.

To ensure that they cook evenly, make sure their sizes are consistent.

Heat up some salted water in a saucepan and simmer for 5 to 7 minutes till the carrot sticks are just soft. *They should be cooked through yet still somewhat crunchy.*

Carrots should be drained and placed aside after cooking.

Get the glaze ready: Melt the butter in a small saucepan over a medium heat.

Mix in the dried culinary lavender flowers and honey and mix well to combine.

Toss the cooked carrots with the honey-lavender glaze in the saucepan to coat the carrots well.

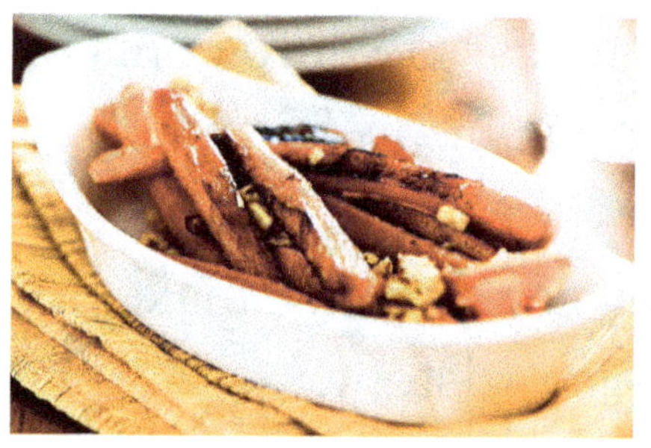

Continue to saute the carrots in the glaze for a further 2 to 3 minutes, stirring now and again until the glaze gradually thickens and covers the carrots.

Add salt and freshly ground black pepper to the glazed carrots and sprinkle some chopped fresh parsley as a garnish if you want to add some more freshness and colour.

Serve the heated glazed carrots as a tasty side dish by transferring them to a serving dish.

PEPPERMINT CHOCOLATE BARK

A tasty and simple-to-make confection, peppermint chocolate bark is ideal for the holidays or any time you're in the mood for something sweet and minty.

Ingredients:

- 12 ounces (340g) of premium black chocolate, chopped
- 12 ounces (340g) of premium white chocolate, chopped
- 1 teaspoon of peppermint essence
- Half a cup of crushed peppermint or candy canes

Instruction:

Use silicone baking mats or parchment paper to line a baking pan.

Melt the white and dark chocolates in separate heatproof basins.

Either use a double boiler or cook in 30-second increments in the microwave, stirring well after each one until the mixture is smooth and melted.

Stir the peppermint essence into the white chocolate once the chocolates have melted.

Using a spatula, evenly distribute the melted dark chocolate into a thin layer on the prepared baking sheet.

Over the top of dark chocolate, drizzle the melted white chocolate.

To obtain a marbled look, carefully stir the two chocolates together using a toothpick or skewer.

While the chocolate is still melted, evenly sprinkle the crushed candy canes or peppermint candies over top.

To ensure the chocolate sets, place the baking sheet in the refrigerator and chill for about 1 hour.

After it has hardened, use a sharp knife or your hands to split the bark into smaller pieces.

Until it's time to serve, keep the peppermint chocolate bark chilled or at room temperature in an airtight container.

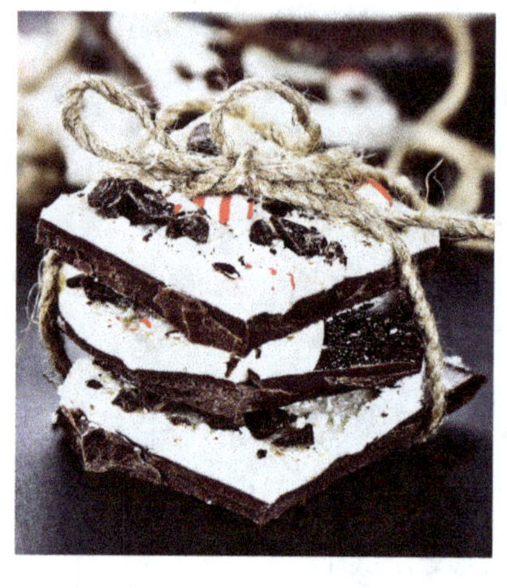

Savour the handmade chocolate bark with peppermint. It's guaranteed to be a hit with friends and family and makes a great present or party favour.

GINGER GARLIC BROCCOLI STIR-FRY

Ingredients:

- 1 large broccoli head, divided into florets
- 3 minced garlic cloves
- 1 tablespoon finely chopped fresh Ginger
- Two tsp soy sauce

- One tablespoon of **optional** Oyster sauce
- One tablespoon of sesame oil
- 1 tablespoon of vegetable oil *(or any other kind of cooking oil)*
- Salt and pepper.
- **Optional**: Sesame seeds as a garnish and Red pepper flakes for heat.

Instruction:

Prepare the Broccoli: Give it a good wash and chop it into little, bite-sized pieces. *If you'd like*, you may also peel and thinly slice the stem.

Get the sauce ready: Combine the sesame oil, oyster sauce *(if using)*, and soy sauce in a small bowl then set aside.

In a large skillet or wok, heat the vegetable oil over medium-high heat.

Add Aromatics: To the heated oil, add the minced ginger and garlic. Stir-fry, taking careful not to burn them - for approximately 30 seconds or until fragrance.

Fill the pan with broccoli florets. Stir-fry the broccoli for 3 to 5 minutes or until it's crisp-tender. *If necessary,* you may cover the pan to assist steam the broccoli for 1 or 2 minutes.

Drizzle the broccoli with the prepared sauce.

To uniformly coat the broccoli with sauce, give it a good stir.

Add salt and pepper to taste, then season and serve. *At this stage,* you may add red pepper flakes if you want it hot.

After mixing everything well, cook for an additional minute.

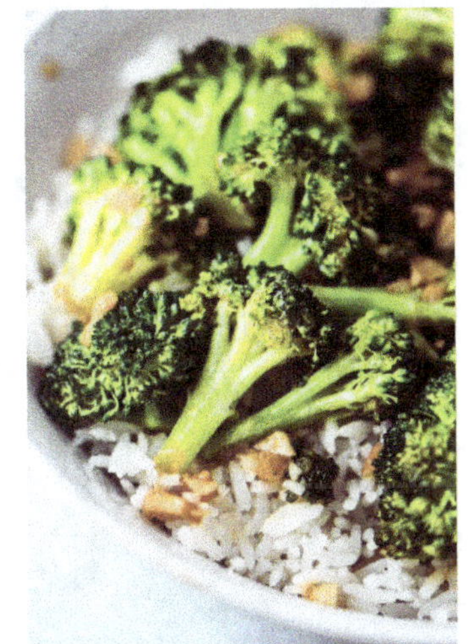

Garnish and Serve:
Take the broccoli off the pan as soon as it's cooked to your preferred softness and the sauce has somewhat thickened.

If desired, sprinkle sesame seeds on top. Serve hot as a main entrée or as a side dish over rice.

BASIL LEMON SORBET

Ingredients:

- 2 cups of water
- 1 cup of sugar, granulated

- One cup of fresh, firmly packed basil leaves
- 1 cup of freshly squeezed lemon juice *(approximately 4-6 lemons)*
- One lemon's zest

Instruction:

Put water and powdered sugar in a saucepan.

Stirring periodically, cook over medium heat until the sugar dissolves completely. *This process will yield simple syrup.*

After the sugar dissolves, turn off the heat source and allow the syrup to come to room temperature.

Wash and blot dry the basil leaves with paper towels as the syrup cools. Take out any rough stems.

Place the cooled simple syrup and basil leaves in a food processor or blender.

Process until the mixture is smooth and the basil is diced finely.

To remove any particles, strain the basil mixture through cheesecloth or a fine mesh sieve into a large dish.

Using a spatula or the back of a spoon, press down on the solids to extract as much liquid as possible.

Incorporate the filtered basil syrup with the lemon zest and fresh lemon juice.

Pour the ingredients into an ice cream machine and process, following the manufacturer's directions, until the consistency of the mixture resembles sorbet. *Usually, it takes twenty to twenty-five minutes.*

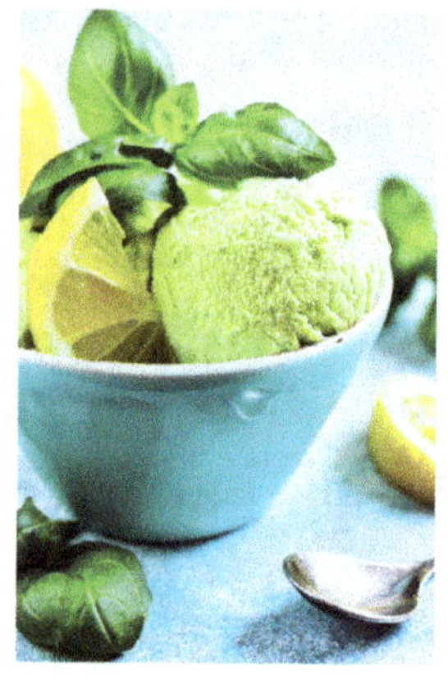

When the sorbet is done, put it in a container that is safe to be frozen and freeze it for at least 4 hours or until it becomes hard.

Allow the sorbet to soften slightly at room temperature for a few minutes before serving.

Enjoy after scooping into bowls or cones.

This cool sorbet of basil and lemon is ideal for a hot summer's day or as a palette cleanser in between dishes.

MILK THISTLE DETOX SMOOTHIE

Ingredients:

- 1 cup of unsweetened almond milk, or any other kind of milk you like.
- 1 ripe banana
- Half a cup of frozen mixed berries, *including raspberries, blueberries and strawberries.*
- One spoonful of flaxseed meal
- One teaspoon of **optional** maple syrup or honey for sweetness.
- 1 tablespoon of milk thistle seeds or 1 teaspoon of powdered milk thistle.
- Grated ginger, 1/2 teaspoon *(optional; adds flavour)*
- One handful of kale or spinach *(optional; adds extra nutrients)*

Instruction: If using milk thistle seeds, use a mortar and pestle or spice grinder to ground them into a fine powder.

Blend together all the ingredients:
To get the right consistency, add more almond milk *if needed* and blend on high until smooth and creamy.

After tasting the smoothie, add additional honey or maple syrup to modify the sweetness *if necessary*.

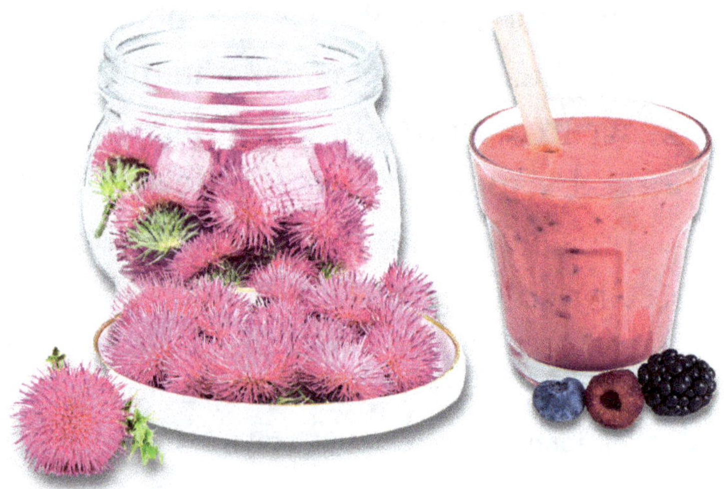

Transfer into glasses and serve right away.

BILBERRY CHIA PUDDING

Ingredients:

- One-fourth cup chia seeds
- One cup of your preferred milk—dairy, almond or coconut.
- 1/4 cup of fresh bilberries *(blueberries work just as well)*
- 1-2 teaspoons of maple syrup or honey, adjusted to taste
- Half a teaspoon of extract from vanilla
- **Extra** fresh bilberries, shredded coconut, sliced almonds or granola are *optional additions*.

Instruction:

Chia seeds and milk should be combined in a jar or mixing dish. Mix well to blend.

Mix in vanilla essence and honey *(or maple syrup)*.

Repeatedly stir until all ingredients are properly combined.

Add the fresh bilberries to the mixture and fold gently. To make a more colourful custard, you may crush some of the bilberries to release their juices.

Refrigerate the bowl or jar for a minimum of 4 hours or better yet, overnight. Cover and store. *This enables the liquid to seep into the chia seeds, creating a pudding-like consistency.*

Stir well to disperse the chia seeds in the chia pudding once it has set.

Serve the chia pudding with bilberries in bowls or jars; garnish with granola, shredded coconut, sliced almonds or more fresh bilberries, *if preferred.*

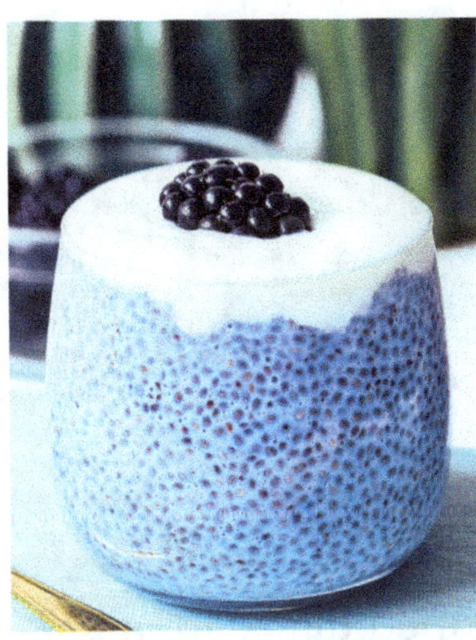

Savour your tasty and nourishing chia pudding with bilberries.

GARLIC HERB SALMON

Ingredients:

- 4 fillets of salmon
- 4 minced garlic cloves
- 2 teaspoons of freshly chopped parsley
- 2 tablespoons of freshly chopped dill

- 2 tablespoons of olive oil
- Salt and pepper.
- slices of lemon for serving

Instruction:

Set oven temperature to 400°F or 200°C.

To prepare the herb combination - combine the minced garlic, olive oil, chopped parsley, chopped dill, salt and pepper in a small bowl.

The salmon fillets should be placed on a baking pan covered with aluminium foil or parchment paper.

Evenly cover the top of each salmon fillet with the herb mixture.

Bake the salmon for 12 to 15 minutes or until it is cooked through and flake readily with a fork, in an oven that has been warmed.

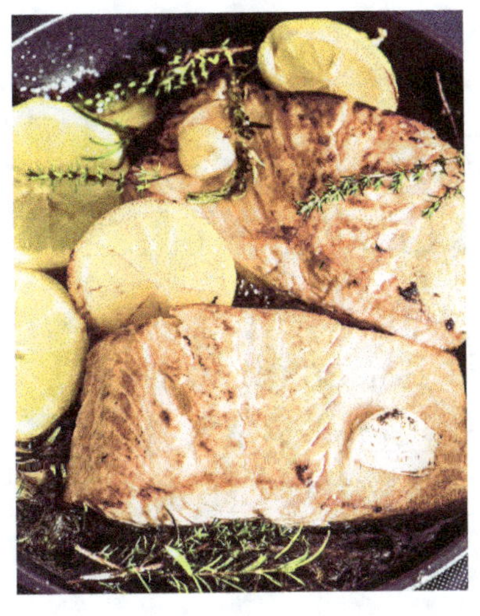

When the salmon is done, take it out of the oven and give it some time to rest.

Warm up the salmon flavoured with garlic and herbs and serve it with lemon wedges for you to squeeze over it.

LEMON VERBENA INFUSED WATER

Ingredients:

- A handful of fresh lemon verbena leaves

- Water *(ideally filtered or spring water)*

Instruction:

To get rid of any dirt or debris, rinse the lemon verbena leaves in cold water.

Roll the leaves in your hands or softly crush them with a spoon to gently bruise them. *Their oils and flavours are released as a result.*

Transfer the crushed lemon verbena leaves to a sanitised glass jar or pitcher. Add enough cold water to the container to cover the leaves.

To enable the flavours to infuse, cover the pitcher or container and let it at room temperature for at least 1 to 2 hours or place it in the refrigerator for the whole night.

After the water has been infused to the appropriate strength, remove the leaves using a strainer.

If preferred, top the cooled lemon verbena-infused water with more lemon verbena leaves or a slice of fresh lemon.

MINT CHOCOLATE AVOCADO MOUSSE

Ingredients:

- Two ripe avocados
- One-fourth cup cocoa powder
- 1/4 cup honey or maple syrup, adjusted to taste
- 1/4 cup milk, either non-dairy or dairy
- Half a teaspoon of extract from peppermint
- A little amount of salt

- Whipped cream, shaved chocolate and mint leaves **are optional** garnishes.

Instruction:

Remove the avocados' flesh with a spoon and transfer it to a food processor or blender.

To the blender, add cocoa powder, milk, peppermint essence, honey or maple syrup and a little teaspoon of salt.

Mix every item until it becomes creamy and smooth.

To make sure everything is properly blended, you may need to pause and scrape along the edges of the blender.

After tasting the mousse, add additional honey, maple syrup or peppermint extract *if necessary* to suit your preferred level of sweetness or mint flavour.

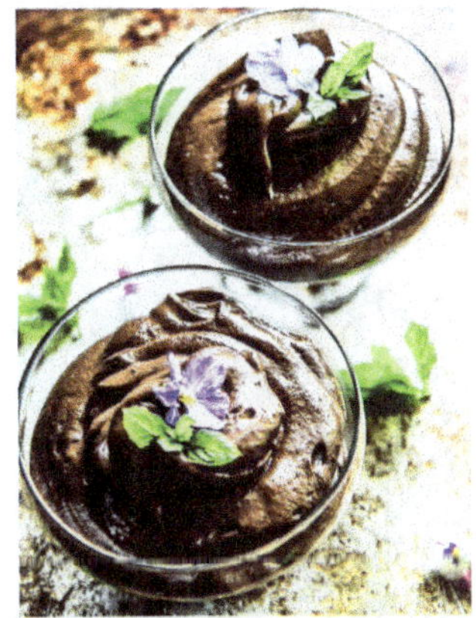

Pour the mousse into glasses or serving bowls once the texture and flavour are to your liking.

To help the mousse firm, chill it in the fridge for at least half an hour.

You may choose to top the mousse with fresh mint leaves, shaved chocolate or a dollop of whipped cream before serving.

In addition to being tasty, this dish is loaded with antioxidants from the cocoa powder and healthy fats from the avocado. This enjoyment is guilt-free.

SAFFRON RICE PILAF

Ingredients:

- One cup of white long-grain rice
- 2 cups broth, either veggie or chicken
- Saffron threads, 1 pinch
- Two teaspoons of olive oil or butter
- 1 little onion, diced finely
- 2 minced garlic cloves
- 1/4 cup of cashews or almonds, chopped (*optional*)
- Salt and pepper.
- Fresh cilantro or parsley chopped for garnish (*optional*)

Instruction:

Till the water runs clear, rinse the rice under cold water. Make sure to drain properly.

Crumble the saffron threads into two teaspoons of heated water or broth in a small dish.

Allow it to soak for 10 to 15 minutes to extract the colour and flavour.

Melt the butter or warm the olive oil in a medium-sized pot over medium heat.

Add the chopped onion and simmer for 3–4 minutes or until transparent.

Once aromatic, add the minced garlic and simmer for an additional 1 to 2 minutes.

Add the rice and simmer, stirring periodically, for 2 to 3 minutes or until the rice is gently toasted.

Pour in the vegetable or chicken broth and the saffron-infused liquid.

To taste, add
salt and pepper
for seasoning.

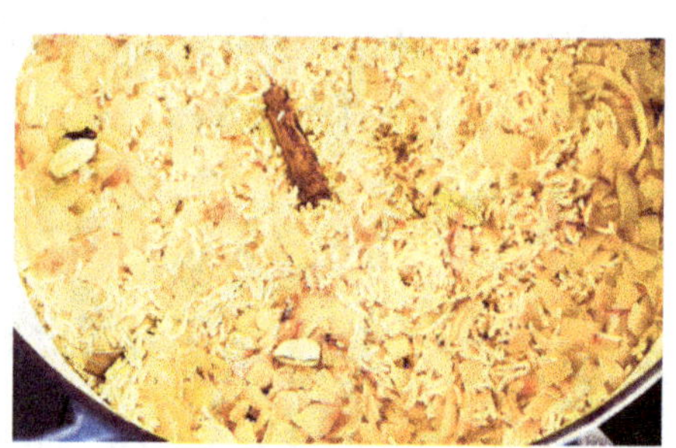

After bringing
the mixture to a boil, turn down the heat.
Once the rice is cooked and the liquid has
been absorbed, simmer it for 15 to 20
minutes with a tightly fitting cover on the
pot.

When the rice is done, use a fork to fluff it
up and add the chopped cashews or
slivered almonds, *if using.*

Before serving, garnish with chopped
cilantro or fresh parsley, *if preferred.*

CAT'S CLAW HERBAL TEA

Native to the Amazon rainforest and other tropical regions of South and Central America, cat's claw (*Uncaria tomentosa*) is a woody vine. Because of its possible health advantages, traditional medicine uses it often.

Please be aware - *however, that herbal medicines have potential negative effects and should be used cautiously since they may interact with drugs.* Before ingesting herbal teas, speak with a healthcare provider, particularly if you have any health issues or concerns.

This is a basic recipe for a herbal tea made from Cat's Claw:

Ingredients:

- 1 Cat's Claw tea bag or 1 teaspoon of dried cat's claw bark
- 1 cup of water
- Taste of honey or lemon *is optional.*

Instruction:

In a small pot or kettle, bring one cup of water to a boil.

Put the tea bag or dried Cat's Claw bark into a cup and pour the boiling water over the tea bag or Cat's Claw bark that is in the cup.

After the cat's claw has steeped in the boiling water for 5 to 10 minutes, cover the cup.

The tea will get stronger the longer it steeps.

Take out the tea bag or Cat's Claw bark from the cup after it has steeped.

If desired, add a squeeze of lemon or honey to the tea to make it sweeter.

Before drinking, give it a good stir and let it cool a little.

Savour your herbal tea and always remember to have it in moderation and seek medical advice if you have any concerns.

CLOVE SPICED BAKED APPLES

Ingredients:

- Four big apples *(Honeycrisp or Granny Smith, for example)*
- One-fourth cup brown sugar

- 1 tsp finely ground cinnamon
- half a teaspoon of powdered cloves
- Two teaspoons of melted butter
- 1/4 cup chopped nuts *(pecans or walnuts, if desired)*
- 1/4 cup dried cranberries or raisins *(optional)*
- Whipped cream or vanilla ice cream, **if desired**, for serving

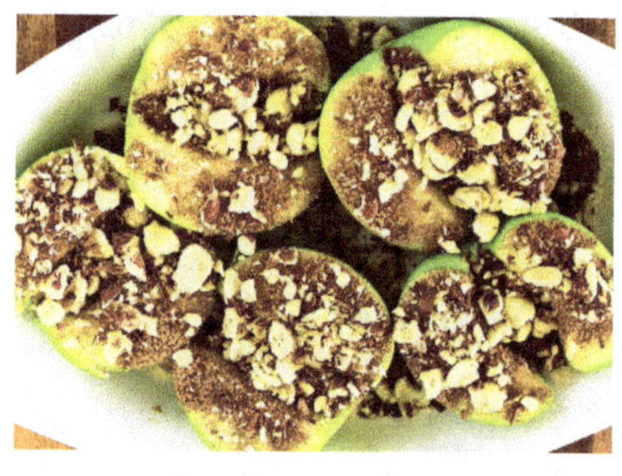

Instruction:

Turn the oven on to 375°F or 190°C.

Grease a baking dish that can accommodate the apples - not too much.

After giving the apples a good cleaning, core them.

The bottoms may be kept whole by removing the cores using an apple corer or a paring knife.

This makes a well for the filling in the middle of each apple.

Combine the ground cloves, ground cinnamon and brown sugar in a small bowl.

Fill the baking dish with the cored apples.

Slice a tiny layer off the bottom of the apples to produce a smooth surface if they don't stand straight on their own.

Melt the butter and combine it with the chopped nuts, raisins or dried cranberries *(if desired)* in a separate dish.

To this bowl, add half of the brown sugar mixture and well combine.

Evenly distribute the buttery mixture among the cored apples by spooning it into their wells.

After the apples are full, sprinkle the leftover brown sugar mixture on top.

Bake the baking dish in the preheated oven for 25 to 30 minutes or until the apples are soft, covered with aluminium foil.

Before serving, take off the foil after baking and let the apples cool for a few minutes.

Warm clove-spiced baked apples may be served plain or with a dollop of whipped cream or a scoop of vanilla ice cream on top, *if preferred.*

GUGGUL LENTIL SOUP

Ingredients:

- 1 cup of dried lentils, any kind
- 4 cups water or vegetable broth
- One tablespoon of oil or ghee
- 1 sliced onion
- 3 minced garlic cloves
- 1 tablespoon of finely chopped ginger
- 1 teaspoon of cumin powder
- 1 tsp finely ground coriander
- ½ a teaspoon of powdered turmeric
- ½ a teaspoon powdered guggul resin
- One chopped carrot
- One chopped celery stalk and one chopped tomato

- Salt to taste.
- To garnish, use fresh cilantro.
- slices of lemon (optional)

Note: **GHEE** – *is a kind of clarified butter from South Asia, is a versatile ingredient that may be utilised in many other types of cooking fats and oils.*

Instruction:

Thoroughly rinse the lentils in cold water until the water becomes clear. After draining, set aside.

Heat the oil or ghee in a big saucepan over medium heat. When the onion is transparent, add it and sauté it for approximately five minutes.

Once aromatic, add the grated ginger and minced garlic to the saucepan and continue to sauté for an additional minute.

Add the guggul resin powder, turmeric powder, powdered cumin and ground coriander and stir, toasting the spices for another minute.

To the saucepan, add the chopped tomato, celery and sliced carrot and cook the veggies for a few minutes until they start to soften while stirring to mix in the spices.

Rinse the lentils and add them to the saucepan along with the vegetable broth or water.

After bringing the soup to a boil, lower the heat, cover it and simmer it for 25 to 30 minutes or until the lentils are soft.

When lentils are cooked, add salt to taste in the soup.

If preferred, top the hot Guggul Lentil Soup with lemon wedges and fresh cilantro.

YARROW SALAD DRESSING

With its earthy, somewhat bitter flavour, yarrow may bring something special to salad dressings.

Ingredients:

- One-fourth cup olive oil
- Two tsp of vinegar made from apple cider
- One tablespoon of maple syrup or honey, adjusted to taste
- One tsp Dijon mustard

- 1-2 teaspoons of freshly cut, finely chopped yarrow flowers and leaves
- Salt and pepper.

Instruction:

Mix the olive oil, apple cider vinegar, honey (*or maple syrup*), and Dijon mustard in a small bowl until well combined.

Finely chop the yarrow flowers and leaves and add them to the dressing mixture.

Depending on how much yarrow flavour you desire, you may change the quantity.

Add salt and pepper to taste, then whisk one more to ensure that everything is combined well.

If needed, taste the dressing and adjust the sweetness or seasoning.

You can either serve it right away over your preferred salad greens or save it for later use in the refrigerator.

Be sure you have accurately identified yarrow before using it in your salad dressing, since there are several plants that seem similar but may be dangerous. If you're not sure how to locate yarrow by foraging, it's usually available in specialised food shops or farmer's markets.

BURDOCK ROOT STIR-FRY

Ingredients:

- 2 to 3 burdock roots, chopped and peeled
- 2 tsp of vegetable oil
- 2 minced garlic cloves
- one tablespoon finely chopped ginger

- 2 julienned carrots
- One bell pepper, cut thinly
- 2 tsp soy sauce
- One-tspn rice vinegar
- One tablespoon sugar or honey, *if desired*
- Salt and pepper.
- Add a garnish of sesame seeds (*optional*).
- Chopped green onions (*optional*) as a garnish

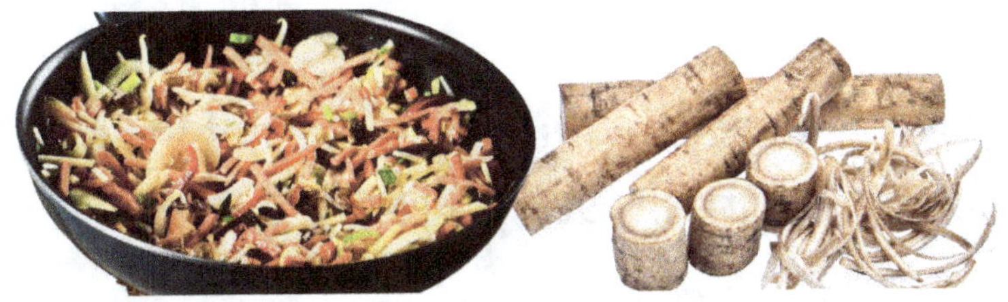

Instruction:

Peel and chop the burdock root into thin strips or julienne slices to prepare it.

To keep the burdock root from browning, put it in a dish of cold water after cutting.

In a large skillet or wok, heat the vegetable oil over medium-high heat.

Add the chopped ginger and garlic to the heated oil and sauté for approximately one minute or until aromatic.

Add the burdock root to the skillet after draining it from the water.

Stir-fry until the burdock root begins to soften, approximately 5 to 7 minutes.

Sliced bell pepper and julienned carrots should be added to the skillet, then stir-fry the veggies for a further 3 to 5 minutes or until they are crisp-tender.

Combine the soy sauce, rice vinegar and honey (*or sugar*) in a small bowl.
After adding the sauce to the stir-fried veggies, mix everything until well covered.

To taste, add salt and pepper for seasoning.

Place the stir-fry on a platter after turning off the heat.

If desired, garnish with chopped green onions and sesame seeds.

Serve hot as a main entrée or as a side dish over rice.

GOAT'S RUE TINCTURE

Ingredients:

- Goat's rue plant, either fresh or dried *(botanical name: Galega officinalis)*
- Strong alcohol *(like brandy or vodka)*

Instruction:

First - give a glass jar a good washing with hot, soapy water, then let it air dry.

Grind or cut the fresh Goat's Rue herb finely if using it - You may use the dried herb just as is.

Spoon the chopped or dried Goat's Rue herb into the glass jar until it is approximately halfway full.

Make sure there are no trapped air bubbles by covering the herb fully with alcohol and cover the jar's lid on securely.

Keep the jar somewhere dark and cold, like a pantry or closet.

For a period of 2 to 4 weeks, gently shake the jar daily to aid in the extraction of the herb's therapeutic qualities into the alcohol.

Once the steeping time is up, strain the liquid to get rid of the herb particles using cheesecloth, a coffee filter or a fine mesh strainer.

Squeeze out as much liquid as you can from the plant stuff.

Pour the resultant tincture into tightly fitting dark glass bottles and put the contents and preparation date on the bottles' labels.

Keep the bottles somewhere cold and dark. Tinctures kept in the right storage may keep for many years.

The right amount of Goat's Rue tincture to use depends on the patient's age, weight, general health and the particular illness they are trying to cure.

For individualised dose recommendations, speaking with a healthcare provider or herbalist is recommended.

Goat's Rue may not work well with certain drugs or health issues. Prior to utilising herbal treatments, always get medical advice, particularly if you are expecting, breastfeeding,, on medication or have a medical condition.

PRICKLY PEAR CACTUS SMOOTHIE

Ingredients:

- One mature, spiny pear cactus fruit
- One frozen banana
- Half a cup of frozen mixed berries, *including blueberries, raspberries and strawberries.*
- Half a cup of dairy-free or plain yoghurt
- 1/2 cup almond milk, unsweetened or any other kind of milk.

- One tablespoon of honey or maple syrup *(optional, depending on desired level of sweetness)*
- Ice cubes—*optional* if you like your smoothie to be colder.

Instruction:

Prepare the fruit of the prickly pear cactus first.

After trimming the fruit's ends with a sharp knife, make a shallow lengthwise incision along one side of the fruit.

Gently remove the skin and throw it away. Chop the fruit flesh into pieces and transfer it to a blender.

To the blender, add the frozen banana, frozen mixed berries, plain yoghurt, almond milk and, **if desired**, honey or maple syrup.

Mix every component until it's smooth. You may adjust the consistency by adding more almond milk if it's too thick.

After tasting the smoothie, add additional honey or maple syrup to modify the sweetness *if necessary*.

To get a cooler smoothie, add a couple of ice cubes to the blender and process until the mixture is smooth once more.

Pour the smoothie into glasses and serve right away *or until it gets the consistency and flavour you like.*

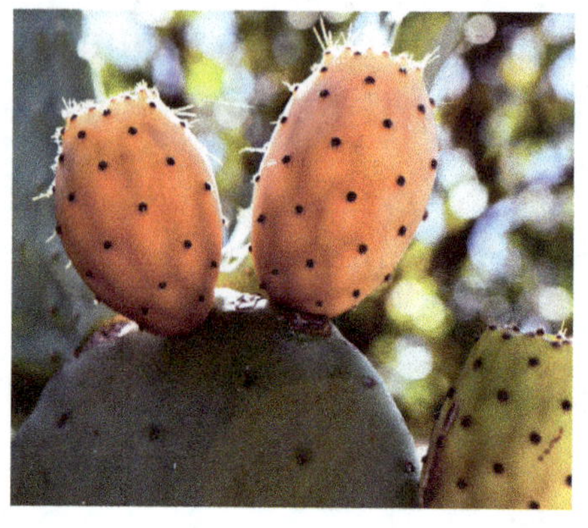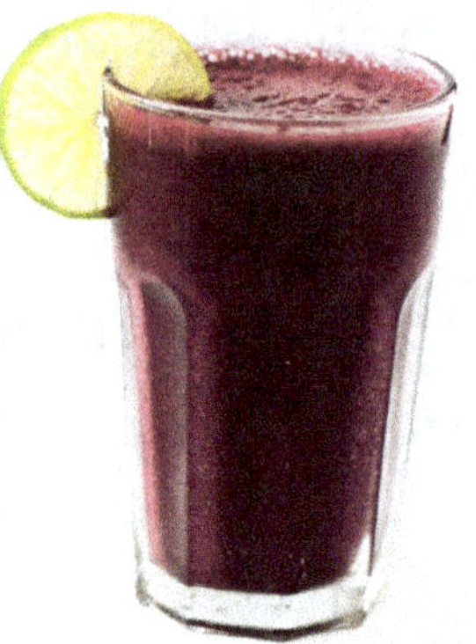

Before serving, you may choose to add some fresh berries or a piece of prickly pear cactus fruit as a garnish to the smoothie.

MISTLETOE INFUSED VINEGAR

Making vinegar infused with mistletoe is a great way to produce a distinctive and celebratory culinary component. This is a basic recipe that you may try:

Ingredients:

- One cup of fresh mistletoe berries and leaves *(make sure they're dirt-free and clean)*
- 2 cups of premium vinegar *(such as champagne, apple cider or white wine vinegar)*

Instruction:

To get rid of any dirt, gently give the berries and mistletoe leaves a gentle washing in cold water.

Using paper towels or a fresh kitchen towel, pat them dry.

You want to use just the soft leaves and berries for the infusion, so remove any tough pieces or stems.

Clean the Jar: Use hot, soapy water to clean a glass jar with a tight-fitting lid.

You may sterilise it by boiling it in water for a short while or you can rinse it well and let it air dry.

Before using, make sure it is thoroughly dry.

Mix the mistletoe with the vinegar:
Fill the sterilised container with the clean mistletoe berries and leaves.

Pour the vinegar in a pot over low heat, warm *(not boiling)* and not hot.

Make sure all of the plant material is immersed by pouring the warm vinegar over the mistletoe in the container.

The Infusion Process: Put the top on the jar firmly.

To let the flavours infuse, keep the jar in a cold, dark area for 2 to 4 weeks. Every few days, you may gently shake the jar to re-distribute the components.

Restricting and Storage: Once the infusion time has passed, pour the vinegar into a sterile, clean container or jar using cheesecloth or a fine-mesh screen.

Throw away the used berries and mistletoe leaves.
Until it's time to use it, carefully seal the bottle and keep it somewhere cold and dark.

Usage: Vinegar infused with mistletoe is a great addition to sauces, marinades, salad dressings and even cocktails and mocktails.

Try a variety of vinegar varieties to get the flavour character you want.

Please note the preparation date on the label of your infused vinegar.

Caution: While eating mistletoe berries or leaves might be harmful, mistletoe is usually regarded as harmless for ornamental use. When handling and cooking mistletoe, make sure you're using the kind meant for culinary use. Before attempting this remedy, think about speaking with an experienced herbalist or medical expert if you have any reservations about using mistletoe.

SIBERIAN GINSENG ENERGY BALLS

Ingredients:

- One cup of oats, rolled

- Half a cup of nut butter, such peanut or almond butter
- 1/4 cup maple syrup or honey
- Two teaspoons of powdered Siberian ginseng
- 1/4 cup of chopped nuts, such cashews, walnuts or almonds.
- 1/4 cup of dried fruit, such as chopped dates, cranberries or raisins
- 1/4 cup of optionally shredded coconut
- One teaspoon of optional vanilla extract
- A dash of salt

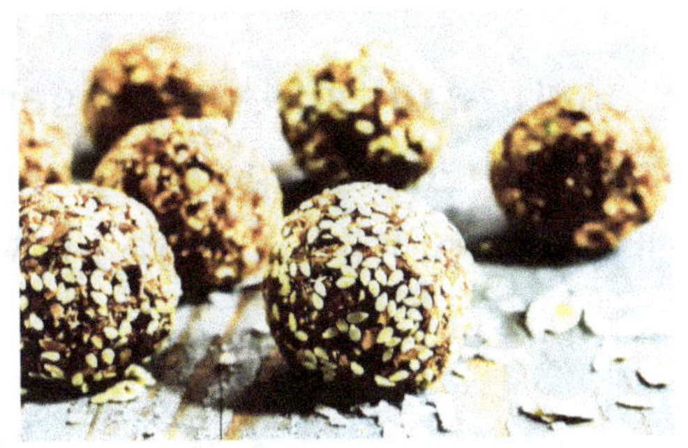

Instruction:

The rolled oats, nut butter, honey or maple syrup, Siberian ginseng powder, chopped nuts, dried fruits, shredded coconut *(if used)*, vanilla essence *(if using)* and a dash of salt should all be combined in a big mixing basin.

Until everything is uniformly incorporated - thoroughly mix.

After the mixture is well mixed, place the bowl in the refrigerator for about half an hour. *It will be simpler to roll the mixture into balls if it is chilled.*

Take the mixture out of the refrigerator when it has chilled. Using your hands, form little parts of the mixture into balls.

You are able to customise them to any desired size.

Arrange the energy balls onto a parchment paper-lined plate or tray.

For additional taste and texture, you may choose to roll the balls in more shredded coconut, chopped almonds or cocoa powder after you've rolled out the whole mixture.

For up to a week, keep the Siberian Ginseng Energy Balls refrigerated in an airtight container.

Savour them as a healthy and convenient snack whenever you need a pick-me-up. You are welcome to change the ingredients to fit your dietary needs or taste preferences.

AMERICAN GINSENG CHICKEN CONGEE

Ingredients:

- 1 cup of rice with jasmine scent
- 6 cups of chicken stock
- One skinless, boneless chicken breast, cut thinly
- 2 slices of root ginseng in America
- 2 ginger slices
- salt to taste.
- **Extra toppings at your discretion:** sliced cooked eggs, green onions, cilantro and mushrooms with sesame oil

Instruction:

Till the water runs clear, rinse the jasmine rice under cold water. Empty the rice.

Heat a large saucepan over medium-high heat and bring the chicken stock to a boil.

Stir well after adding the rinsed jasmine rice to the boiling stock.

After lowering the heat to low, simmer the rice for approximately 30 minutes, stirring now and again to avoid sticking or until the rice has broken down and the congee has thickened.

As the congee simmers, get the chicken ready. Sprinkle salt on the chicken breast slices that are very thin.

Heat a little amount of oil in a different pan over medium-high heat.

After adding the sliced chicken breast, simmer it for 5 to 7 minutes or until it is done and has a golden brown hue then set aside.

Add the cooked chicken pieces, ginger slices and American ginseng root slices to the pot after the congee has thickened.

Mix well to blend.

To help the flavours combine, boil the congee for a further 10 to 15 minutes.

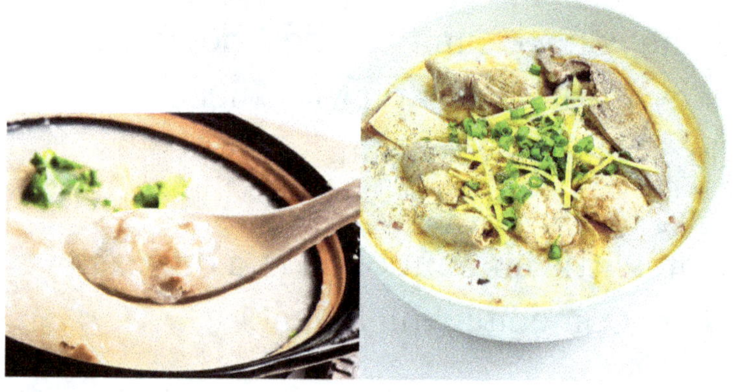

If needed, add more salt to the seasoning after tasting the congee.

Serve the congee hot, topped with cooked eggs, sliced green onions, cilantro and, *if preferred,* a drizzle of sesame oil.

HAWTHORN BERRY COMPOTE

Ingredients:

- 2 cups freshly cleaned and stemmed hawthorn berries
- one-fourth cup water
- 1/4 cup sugar or honey, *depending on taste*
- 1 tsp lemon juice
- ½ a teaspoon of cinnamon, *if desired*

Instruction:

Get the berries ready: To get rid of any dirt or debris, rinse the hawthorn berries under cold water.

Remove the stems and discard any berries that are broken or bruised.

Put the hawthorn berries and water in a saucepan. Over medium heat, bring the mixture to a moderate simmer.

After the berries begin to soften, turn down the heat to a low simmer and let them for 10 to 15 minutes, stirring now and again - *the berries need to disintegrate and release their liquid contents.*

Sweeten: Stir the berries while they are cooking and add honey or sugar, making sure it melts

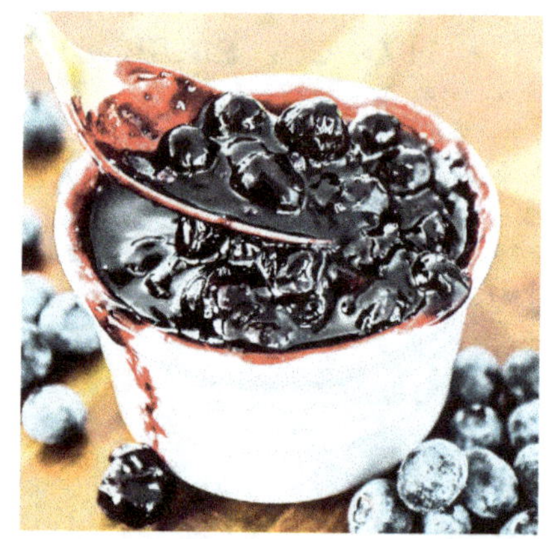

thoroughly. You may adjust the sweetness to suit your taste.

Add the cinnamon (*if using*) and lemon juice for flavour. The cinnamon adds depth and warmth, while the lemon juice lends a crisp acidity.

Thicken (optional): If you'd like your compote to have a little more thickness, you may use a potato masher or fork to crush some of the berries to release some of their natural pectin.

As an alternative, you might make a slurry with a tiny quantity of cornflour or arrowroot powder and whisk it into the compote.

Simmer for a further 2 to 3 minutes or until the compote begins to slightly thicken.

To serve, take the compote from the stove and allow it to cool a little bit. It may be served warm or cold, according to your own choice.

 You can keep any leftover compote in the fridge for up to a week by storing it in an airtight container.

Savour the handmade compote made with hawthorn berries. Serve it over toast, yoghurt, muesli or pancakes for a wonderful treat.

GINGERBREAD CHIA SEED PUDDING

Ingredients:

- 1/4 cup of chia seeds.
- One cup of milk, either dairy-free or plant-based *(such almond or coconut milk)*.
- One spoonful of honey or maple syrup

- ½ a teaspoon of ginger powder
- ½ a teaspoon of cinnamon powder
- 1/4 teaspoon of ground nutmeg
- 1/4 tsp ground cloves
- ½ a teaspoon of extract from vanilla
- **Optional garnishes** include chopped nuts, dried cranberries, whipped cream and almond slices.

Instruction:

Chia seeds, milk, maple syrup or honey, ground ginger, ground cinnamon, ground nutmeg, ground cloves and vanilla essence should all be combined in a dish or container.

Toss to thoroughly mix in all the ingredients.

Refrigerate the jar or dish for a minimum of 2 hours or overnight - covered. This

To uniformly distribute the chia seeds, give the custard a thorough stir once it has set.

Serve the cooled gingerbread chia seed pudding with your preferred toppings such as - chopped nuts, dried cranberries, whipped cream or sliced almonds.

Savour your tasty and nutritious chia seed pudding with gingerbread.

MOMORDICA CHARANTIA JUICE

Momordica charantia, sometimes referred to as bitter melon or bitter gourd, is a tropical vine that is extensively grown for its fruit, which is said to provide a number of health advantages.

Juice from bitter melon is often ingested for possible health benefits, especially in controlling blood sugar levels. Below's a quick recipe to make juice from Momordica charantia -

Ingredients:

- 1 bitter, medium-sized melon
- 1 to 2 teaspoons of honey or any other preferred sweetener (to taste)
- One or two glasses of water
- Cubes of ice (optional)

Instruction:

Under running water, give the bitter melon a thorough wash.

Using a spoon, remove the seeds and pith from the bitter melon after slicing it lengthwise. The pith and seeds may be thrown away or saved for use in other recipes.

To make mixing simpler, chop the bitter melon into smaller pieces.

Put the slices of bitter melon in a blender and add one or two glasses of water.

Depending on how concentrated you want the juice to be, adjust the water quantity. *If necessary*, add extra water after starting with less.

Blend the mix until it's smooth. To make sure all the parts are well combined, you may need to stop and scrape down the sides of the blender.

Taste the mixture when it's smooth. You may add 1 or 2 teaspoons of honey or any other preferred sweetener, if you find it to be too harsh and then toss to blend again.

To get rid of any pulp or particles, strain the juice using cheesecloth or a fine mesh strainer.

If you would rather have a thicker, higher-fibre juice, you may skip this step.

If preferred, pour the strained juice into a glass and top with ice cubes.
Before serving, stir the liquid and enjoy.

While some people feel that a hint of sweetness makes bitter melon juice more tolerable, others prefer to drink it that way in order to completely appreciate its inherent bitterness. You may adjust the sweetness to suit your taste. For extra taste and health advantages, you may also alter this recipe by adding additional ingredients like ginger or lemon juice.

ECHINACEA IMMUNE BOOSTING SOUP

Ingredients:

- One tablespoon of olive oil
- One chopped onion
- 3 minced garlic cloves
- Diced 2 carrots
- 2 celery stalks - Diced
- 1 cup finely chopped spinach or greens
- 1 cup of canned or fresh diced tomatoes
- Six cups of vegetable stock
- 1 teaspoon of dried echinacea or 2–3 tea bags of echinacea
- Salt and pepper.

* For garnish, use fresh parsley *(optional)*.

Instruction:

In a big saucepan, warm up the olive oil over medium heat. Add minced garlic and chopped onion.

Sauté for 3–4 minutes or until onions are transparent and garlic is aromatic.

Add the chopped celery and carrots to the saucepan and cook for another 5 minutes, stirring now and again.

Then add the diced tomatoes and veggie broth. After bringing the soup to a boil, lower the heat and simmer it for 15 to 20 minutes or until the veggies are soft.

In the meanwhile, create a sachet or infuser by tying dried echinacea in a tiny piece of cheesecloth.

To the soup pot, add the sachet of Echinacea tea bags straight into the pot *if you're using them.*

After adding the chopped spinach or kale, simmer for a further 5 minutes then take out the tea bags or sachet of echinacea from the broth.

To taste, add salt and pepper for seasoning.

If preferred, top the soup with fresh parsley after ladling it into bowls.

Serve and enjoy your immune-stimulating Echinacea soup hot.

Modify the ingredients and spices to suit your tastes. Not only is this soup tasty, but the veggies and echinacea provide a wealth of immune-boosting minerals.

FENUGREEK SEED BREAD

Ingredients:

- 1 cup all-purpose flour
- 2 cups whole wheat flour
- 1 tablespoon fenugreek seeds
- One tsp of dried active yeast
- One tablespoon of sugar or honey,
- One teaspoon of salt
- 1 ¼ cups heated water
- 2 tsp olive oil

Instruction:

Activate the yeast: Melt sugar *(or honey)* in a small basin of heated water. After adding the yeast to the water, let it rest for 5 to 10 minutes or until it foams.

Get the dough ready:
Mix together the fenugreek seeds, salt, whole wheat flour and all-purpose flour in a large mixing basin.

Create a well in the middle and add the olive oil and active yeast mixture and stir to make a dough.

After transferring the dough to a floured surface, knead it for 8 to 10 minutes or until it becomes elastic and smooth.

The dough can be overly sticky, in which case you might need to add a little more flour.

After putting the dough in a greased bowl and covering it with plastic wrap or a fresh kitchen towel, let it rise in a warm location until it has doubled in size, which should take one to 1 ½ hours.

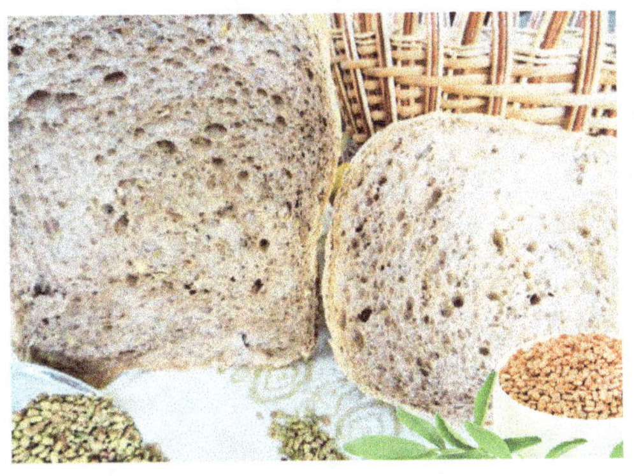

Form the Loaf: To release the air bubbles in the rising dough, punch it down. Form it into a loaf and put it in a loaf pan that has been oiled.

Second Rising: After putting a fresh kitchen towel or plastic wrap over the loaf pan, let it rise once more for 30 to 45 minutes or until it has doubled in size.

Set the oven temperature to 375°F or 190°C, in the last 15 minutes of the second rise.

After the dough has risen, bake the bread for approximately 30 to 35 minutes in a preheated oven or until the bottom of the loaf sounds hollow when you tap it and the crust is golden brown.

Chill and Serve:

Once the bread is taken out of the oven, it should cool in the pan for a few minutes before being transferred to a wire rack to finish cooling. Slice and serve.

HIBISCUS GINGER ICED TEA

Ingredients:

- Four cups of water
- 1/4 cup of hibiscus blossoms, dried
- A 2-inch piece of freshly sliced ginger and 2 to 3 tablespoons of honey or your preferred sweetener *(adjust to taste)*
- Cubes of ice
- For garnish, use *optional* mint leaves or slices of lemon.

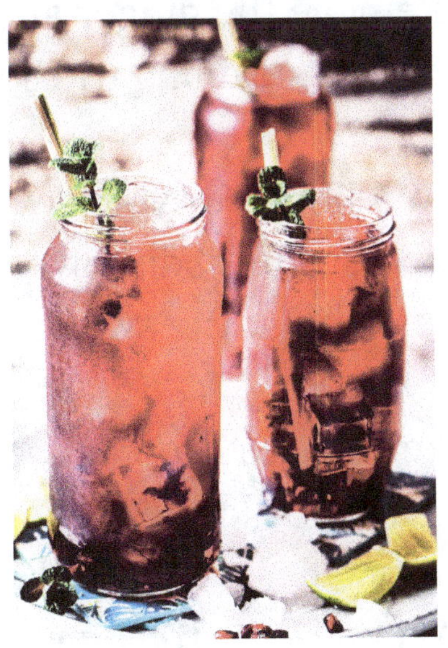

Instruction:

Heat the water in a pot until it boils.

When the water reaches a boiling point, turn off the heat and stir in the sliced ginger and dried hibiscus flowers.

Allow the flavours to permeate by steeping the mixture for around 15-20 minutes.

Remove the ginger and hibiscus blossoms before straining the liquid into a pitcher.

Add honey or your favourite sweetener and stir until dissolved. *If necessary,* taste and adjust the sweetness.

Let the tea drop to room temperature by chilling it in the refrigerator.

When ready to serve, place ice cubes in glasses and cover the ice with the cooled hibiscus ginger tea.

If desired, garnish with mint leaves or slices of lemon. Before serving, give your Hibiscus Ginger Iced Tea a little stir and enjoy.

OKRA STIR-FRY

Ingredients:

- 1 pound of freshly cleaned and trimmed okra
- 2 tsp of vegetable oil
- 2 minced garlic cloves
- One little onion, chopped
- One bell pepper, chopped
- One tsp soy sauce
- One tsp of sesame oil
- Salt and pepper.
- For more heat, feel free to add hot sauce or chilli flakes.

- Chopped cilantro or green onions are an *optional garnish.*

Instruction:

Cut off the ends of the okra and cut it into 1/2-inch pieces.
In a large skillet or wok, heat the vegetable oil over medium-high heat.

In the pan, add the minced garlic and the sliced onions. Sauté for 2 to 3 minutes or until the onions become transparent and aromatic.

After adding the sliced bell pepper to the pan, sauté it for a further 2 to 3 minutes or until it starts to soften.

Add the sliced okra to the pan and stir-fry it for approximately 5 to 7 minutes till when the okra is soft but still somewhat crunchy.

Add salt, pepper, sesame oil and soy sauce to the stir-fry to season it.

At this time, you may also add chilli flakes or hot sauce if you want it spicy.

Stir-fry for a further 2 to 3 minutes or until everything is thoroughly cooked and well mixed.

If necessary, taste and adjust the seasoning. *If desired,* garnish with chopped cilantro or green onions.

Serve hot as a main entrée or as a side dish over cooked rice.

SOYBEAN HUMMUS

Ingredients:

- One can (15 oz) of washed and drained soybeans
- One-fourth cup tahini
- 2 minced garlic cloves
- 1/4 cup of freshly squeezed lemon juice
- Two tsp olive oil
- ½ a teaspoon of cumin powder
- Salt to taste.
- Water *(as required to get the right consistency)*
- **Garnishes optional**: sesame seeds, minced parsley, paprika and olive oil

Instruction:

Add the soybeans, tahini, lemon juice, cumin, olive oil and a dash of salt to a food processor.

Using a food processor scrape down the sides as necessary - blend the items until they are smooth.

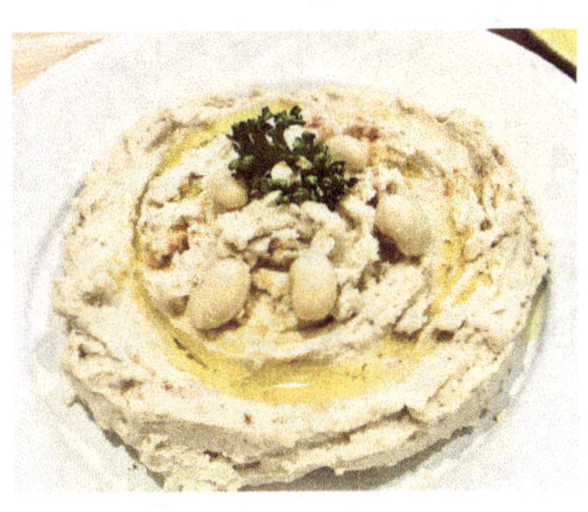

Add water a tablespoon at a time to the mixture if it's too thick until you have the right consistency.

After tasting the hummus, adjust the seasoning by adding extra lemon juice or salt as necessary.

Move the hummus to a serving dish after it has the flavour and consistency you want.

If you'd like, top the hummus with a little olive oil and garnish with sesame seeds, chopped parsley or paprika.

Serve the soybean hummus with your preferred dipping sauces, crackers, pita bread or sliced veggies.

ASTRAGALUS CHICKEN BONE BROTH

Ingredients:

- One whole organic chicken carcass, including the skin, bones and any remaining flesh.
- 2 to 3 astragalus root pieces
- 1 onion
- two quartered Carrots
- two chopped celery stalks
- 4 chopped garlic cloves - crushed
- 1 spoonful of vinegar made from apple cider
- 1 tsp full peppercorns

- 2 bay leaves
- Salt to taste in water *(optional)*
- As a garnish, fresh parsley is **optional.**

Instruction:

Give the chicken carcass a quick rinse in cold water and transfer it to a large stockpot or slow cooker.

To the saucepan, add the astragalus root, onion, peppercorns, bay leaves, carrots, celery and garlic.

Add enough water to the saucepan to cover each item by a few inches.

The broth should be brought to a boil over high heat, then simmered for at least 4–6 hours *(or up to 24 hours for optimum flavour and nutrient extraction)* with a partly covered lid.

150

If you're using a slow cooker, cook it for 8 to 10 hours on low heat.

Using a ladle or spoon, skim any froth or particles that come to the top of the simmering soup.

When the broth is done boiling, take the saucepan off of the hob and let it cool a little.

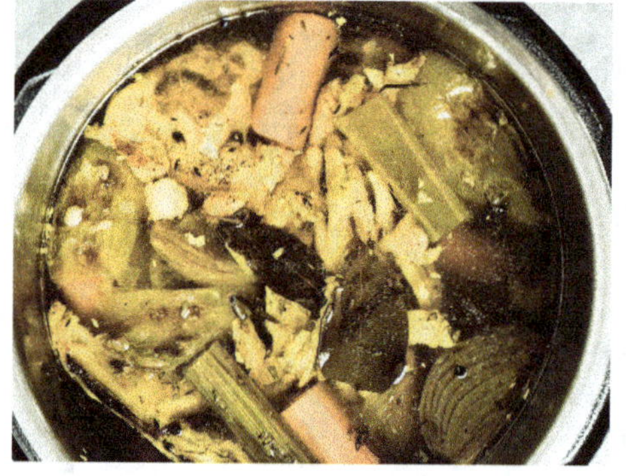

To get rid of the particles, strain the broth into a clean container using cheesecloth or a fine-mesh sieve. Throw away the solids.

If desired, add salt to taste and season the broth.

The broth may be frozen for extended storage or kept in the fridge for up to five days.

If desired, top the hot dish with freshly chopped parsley and reheat the broth as required.

RHODIOLA ROSEA TEA

Ingredients:

- One teaspoon *(or one tablespoon, if using fresh root)* of dried Rhodiola rosea
- One cup of water
- Lemon or honey *(optional; adds flavour)*

Instruction:

Fill a saucepan or kettle with one cup of boiling water.
Put the dried root of Rhodiola rosea in a heat-resistant cup or teapot.

Cut the fresh Rhodiola Rosea root into little pieces before putting it in the cup or teapot.

Pour the water over the Rhodiola Rosea root in the teapot or cup after it reaches a roaring boil.

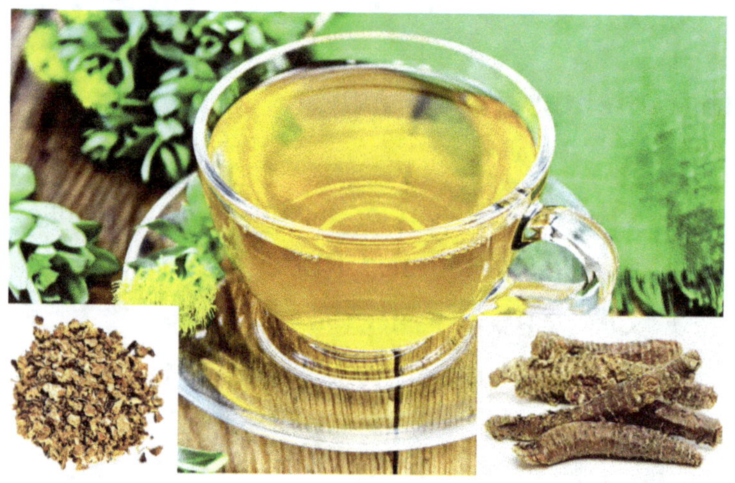

Allow the Rhodiola Rosea root to soak in the hot water for 10 to 15 minutes, covered with a saucer or lid on the teapot. *This permits the good chemicals to seep into the water.*

Strain the tea to get rid of the bits of
Rhodiola Rosea root once it has steeped.

If desired, add a squeeze of lemon or honey
to the tea to make it sweeter.
While the tea is still warm, thoroughly stir
it and enjoy.

Prior to ingesting Rhodiola Rosea tea, always get
medical advice, particularly if you have any
underlying medical issues or are already taking
medication.

ASHWAGANDHA GOLDEN MILK LATTE

Warm and calming, the Ashwagandha
Golden Milk Latte blends the health
benefits of ashwagandha with the
reassuring tastes of turmeric and spices.

Ingredients:

- One cup of milk *(vegan or dairy, such as oat, almond or coconut milk)*
- one tsp finely ground turmeric
- ½ a teaspoon of cinnamon powder
- 1/4 tsp ground ginger
- 1/4 teaspoon of cardamom powder
- 1/4 tsp ground black pepper
- One tsp honey or maple syrup *(add or subtract according to taste)*
- 1 ½ tsp ashwagandha powder
- ½ a teaspoon of optional vanilla essence

Instruction:

The milk should be heated in a small saucepan over medium heat until it begins to steam. *Take care not to allow it to boil.*

In a small bowl, combine the ashwagandha powder, cardamom, ginger,

cinnamon and black pepper; set aside
while the milk heats.

When the milk begins to steam, stir in the
spice blend until well mixed.

To let the flavours merge together, cook
the milk mixture for a further 2 to 3
minutes while stirring from time to time.

If adding maple syrup or honey, mix it in
until it dissolves.

Take the pot off of the burner and, *if using,*
whisk in the vanilla essence.

Transfer the warm golden milk latte into a
cup.

Serve your warming and filling Golden
Milk Latte with ashwagandha - To suit

your taste, adjust the spices and
sweetness.

CHASTE TREE BERRY SMOOTHIE

The berry of the chaste tree, sometimes called Vitex agnus-castus, is occasionally used in herbal remedies.

It's important to remember that its safety for ingestion might vary based on a number of circumstances, including a person's medical history and possible drug interactions. *Before using any herbal product, including chaste tree berry, always get medical advice.*

I wouldn't advise using chaste tree berry in a smoothie recipe because of the possible issues with it. Alternatively, I can offer you this delicious and nourishing smoothie recipe that doesn't use chaste tree berries:

SMOOTHIE BERRY BLAST

Ingredients:

- One cup of mixed berries, including raspberries, blueberries and strawberries.
- One ripe banana
- Half a cup of Greek yoghurt *(vegan options might use dairy-free yoghurt)*
- Half a cup of kale or spinach leaves *(optional for extra nutrition)*
- Half a cup of almond milk or any other kind of milk.
- 1 tablespoon of optionally sweetened maple syrup or honey
- **(Optional, for a cooler smoothie)** Ice cubes

Instruction:

Peel the banana and wash the berries. Fill a blender with all of the ingredients. Process at high speed until creamy and smooth.

Taste and add extra honey or maple syrup to adjust sweetness if needed.

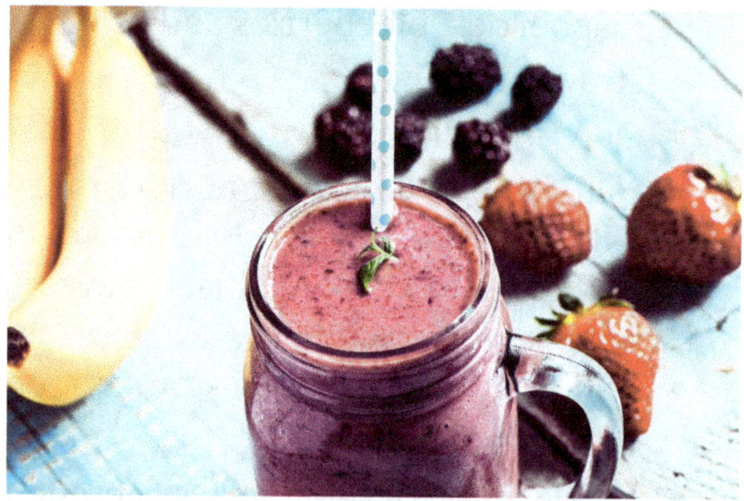

To get the right consistency, thin down any extra almond milk or water if the smoothie is too thick.

Transfer into glasses and serve right away.

LICORICE ROOT HERBAL INFUSION

It's easy to make a herbal infusion using licorice root with only a few components. The naturally sweet flavour of licorice root is accompanied by a host of health advantages. This is a simple method for making a herbal infusion made from licorice root:

Ingredients:

- 1 tablespoon of licorice root, dried
- 2 cups of water

- **Optional**: For flavouring, use lemon or honey *(if desired)*

Instruction:

In a pot or kettle, first bring two cups of water to a boil.

After the water reaches a boiling point, turn down the heat to a low setting and stir in 1 tablespoon of dried licorice root.

Allow the licorice root to steep in the boiling water for 5 to 10 minutes by placing a cover on the pot or kettle.

Depending on how intense you want the flavour to be, you may adjust the steeping time.

Remember that if you soak licorice root for an extended period of time, it might become bitter, so keep an eye on it.

After the licorice root pieces have steeped, take the pot or kettle from the burner and filter the liquid – *For this stage, you may use a tea infuser or a strainer with fine mesh.*

To serve, transfer the infusion of licorice root into mugs or glasses. You may have it just the way it is or you can add honey or lemon to taste if you'd want it sweeter or tangier.

Optional: To improve the flavour of your licorice root infusion, feel free to experiment with other herbs or spices – Peppermint, cinnamon and ginger are a few typical additives.

You can have it hot or cold, according to your own inclination. Not everyone should take licorice root, particularly if they have high blood pressure or other medical issues.

CONCLUSION

To sum up, herbal therapies provide a potential way to help with Type 2 Diabetes control. They may supplement current medications by possibly enhancing insulin sensitivity, controlling blood sugar levels and reducing some of the related problems, even if they might not completely replace traditional treatments.

Still, it's essential to proceed cautiously while using herbal medicines because of the possibility of drug interactions and

the fact that individual effectiveness
varies.

To create standardised doses, guarantee
safety and prove their efficacy - further
investigation and clinical studies are
required. Under the supervision of
medical experts.

Including herbal medicines into a
complete treatment plan has the potential
to improve the quality of life for those
with diabetes and to improve overall
diabetes control.

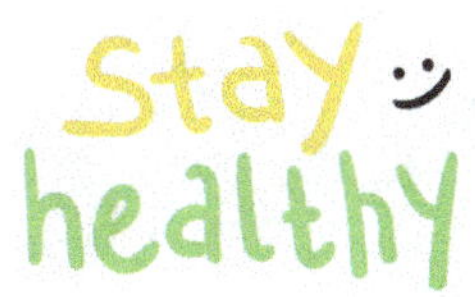